More

Shibari

You Can *Use*

Passionate Rope Bondage
and Intimate Connection

More Shibari **You Can *Use***

Passionate Rope Bondage and Intimate Connection

By **Lee Harrington**

Photography by **RiggerJay**

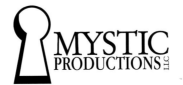

MYSTIC PRODUCTIONS LLC

Notice

Personal responsibility is a basic tenet of adult activity. Like any adult activity, rope bondage inherently contains risk of both physical and emotional injury. Any information or safety guidelines provided in this book are solely suggestions on ways to help reduce those inherent risks. By deciding to engage in any adult activity, including those detailed in this book, you are taking on physical and emotional responsibility for your own actions, and agree to hold harmless all individuals associated with the creation, publication and sale of this book.

All text and rope work by Lee Harrington
www.PassionAndSoul.com

All photography by RiggerJay
www.RiggerJay.com

Book cover and layout design by Rob River
www.RobRiver.com

ISBN 978-0-9778727-5-6
Ebooks: MOBI — 978-0-9778727-3-2
               ePub — 978-0-9778727-4-9
               PDF — 978-0-9778727-9-4

Dedicated to Ayem Willing
    who connected with intention
and will stay forever in our hearts.

Table of Contents

Introduction

Though it is fascinating to learn about the modern styles of Japanese-inspired rope bondage evolving through performance and intimate exploration internationally, that is likely not why you picked up this book. You picked it up because you are interested in the ideas of restraint, beauty, erotic connection, or sexy delight. You want to be bound by, or bind, your lover. You want to explore, learn, and make magic happen.

And you can!

Whether you are hungry for more information after reading *Shibari You Can Use: Japanese Rope Bondage and Erotic Macramé,* have been exploring rope for years, or are enjoying rope bondage for the first time, this is the book for you.

Just as the first Shibari book is known for its easy step-by-step directions, More Shibari will follow the clear directional style of its sibling. It even includes some of the silliness the old book had, because playfulness can help a lot of us learn. However, instead of stopping after a tie is done or applied in basic forms, this book will continue forward into various exercises. These are additional ideas on how to use the tie and connect with a partner by using it. This is important because when we are learning new ties, we sometimes get so sucked into the new technique that we can forget about the passion and connection that brought us to rope in the first place.

So, are you ready to get tying? Ready to learn simple cuffs, create practical and decorative chest harnesses, and bind faces? Does crafting gags, crotch ropes, and speed bondage get you going? Are you excited about incorporating power exchange with your bondage? Delighted that the exercises in the book will help you work on connecting with your partner, not just your rope? Fantastic—you're in the right place.

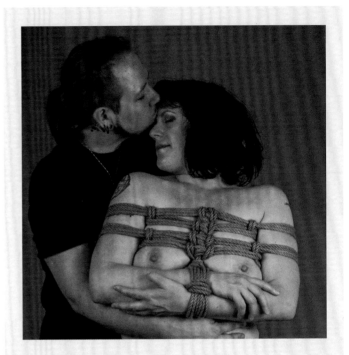

Rope for passion, rope for connection, rope demystified.

This book is not meant for your bookshelf, to gather dust and only be pulled out for titillation value (though feel free to be titillated!). It was designed to play with, engage with, and help you connect with your partner(s). It's meant to be flipped open and consulted, shoved in your toy bag, and shared with friends. Make notes or sketches in the margins if that grabs you. Use it for what you authentically are called to do. Get excited.

Then take that excitement, and let's explore... More Shibari You Can Use!

Purpose and Passion

We are called to rope bondage for a thousand different reasons. Why we are into rope or restraint can dramatically affect our choices of the ties and poses we play with.

But that's not all. Our purpose determines how long we will engage in a scene, the type of rope we will use, and even the wardrobe (or lack thereof) we will wear. Our "whys" allow us to understand where we are coming from, where our partners are coming from, and each of our needs, wants and desires.

The reasons individuals are drawn to rope are myriad, including but not limited to:

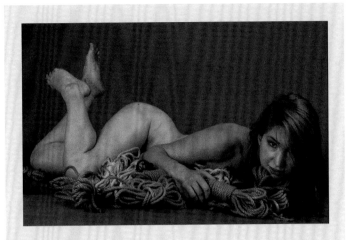

If your partner is into rope, that might be enough of a reason to explore bondage.

- Restraint
- Sensuality
- Fun
- Trust
- Beauty
- Excitement
- Naughtiness
- Struggling
- Experimentation
- Dominance
- Fetish Play
- Connection
- Sacredness
- Sex Positions
- Firmness
- Softness
- Endurance
- Submission
- Playing Dress-Up
- Partner's Interest
- Ferocity
- Desire
- Teasing
- Pain
- Silliness
- Contortion
- Being Artistic
- Tantra
- Touch
- Playfulness
- Sexy Photos
- Taboo
- Something New
- Yoga/Stretching
- Performance
- Exhibitionism
- Suffering
- Tactile Experience
- Role-Playing
- Feeling Pretty

There is no right reason to be into bondage. As a pair of individuals (or triad, or group of friends) exploring rope, you will likely have a variety of reasons you want to tie or be tied. Maybe your reasons today are different than what your reason will be tomorrow. It is important to know not only why you are into rope, but why your partner is as well.

Communicating Desires

Communicating what we are into, our desires, our limits, our concerns, and our delights is referred to cumulatively as "negotiation." Styles of negotiation can include:

- Curling up in bed and sharing fantasies
- Looking at pornography together and letting each other know what turns you on
- Examining someone's erotic "toy bag" and asking questions
- Sending notes or pictures back and forth over the internet
- Having a phone conversation... or twenty
- Filling out a negotiation form/checklist (either to help you figure out your own desires, or to share the form with a partner)
- Discussing your interests over a nice dinner or coffee
- Attending classes and talking about what you are each into, then asking questions of each other afterwards
- and more!

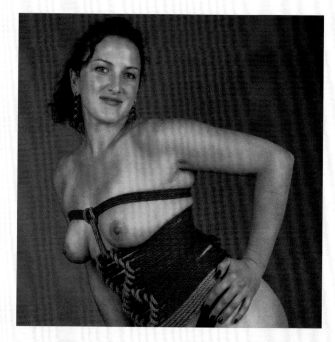

Quick-style corsets (page113)

Let's say two players share their desires with one another. One says they are turned on by speed bondage, and the other says they are delighted by being made beautiful. Does that mean they aren't compatible? Not at all. It means that they, as a pair, get to explore combination possibilities such as some of the ideas shown here on these two pages.

Staying open and creative helps us find something that works for everyone.

If your partner says that an image or concept is interesting to them, there are many types of responses you can have. Responses to someone that gain more information (rather than making assumptions) include:

- Thank you for sharing that with me.
- What about that appeals to you?
- Would you be interested to doing something like that with me?

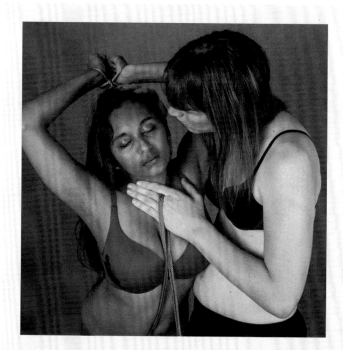

Texas handcuff (page 36) pulled up through the crotch

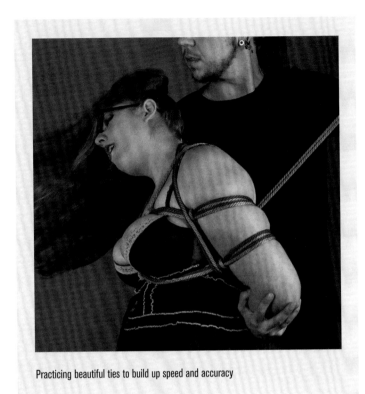

Practicing beautiful ties to build up speed and accuracy

Being able to say you enjoy the notion of sensual rope because it would allow you a chance to be present and connect with your beloved might help them understand your interests. You might just be running into the projections other people have about what they think bondage (or that type of bondage) is about. There are some individuals who associate bondage with abuse or negative media representations rather than consensual passion, beauty or fun. Sharing your wishes, as well as what you are not interested in, from a place of compassionate communication can help build intimacy and trust.

Remember that sharing our fantasies is not the same thing as demanding activities or placing guilt and blame on our partners. Just because you have asked for a specific type of activity does not mean your partner should be required to do that activity—everyone needs to freely consent to the activities involved. Fully engaged consent is not just about "not saying no." It is about sharing an enthusiastic yes! And just because someone says they fantasized about something, or wanted to do something on the day they first talked about it, does not mean it is what they want to do today. Make sure to check in to make sure everyone is on the same page before playing.

- What about that turns you on?
- What might that look like for you/us?
- Please tell me more.

Inter-personal connection is aided through these sorts of energetically open questions, presented in a loving tone, as compared to statements such as:

- That is so strange.
- Who would like that?
- What is wrong with you?
- You're kidding, right?

The first category helps engage and ally with our partners. The second might shut them down, making them wary of sharing more about their desires—they do not help construct open and loving dialogue.

Exploring language and ideas in advance such as why you like rope, or what kinds of play appeals to you, can help a dialogue be more successful as well.

Beyond all of the words, our body shares a lot of information. Consider negotiating with someone who you know is already into bondage by sharing passions through the flesh. Consensually bind a lover's wrist to see if they respond with a smile, or grinding hips. Getting this sort of information is a valid form of negotiation, as long as it is clear in advance that everyone has consented to, and agreed upon, this style of information sharing. An enthusiastic yes is a must.

This sort of information sharing also includes the body language involved when our partners tell us their desires. Watching for additional information through their eyes, lips, body adjustments, heartbeat, and perspiration offers the chance to communicate further information. Combining words with our bodily passions can help give us the best of both worlds, while also confirming that our "hunches" are correct.

Communicating During Play

Wait! Don't I have to have a safeword and have signed waivers before we do bondage? Safewords can be a good idea, especially if engaging in fantasy role-playing scenarios. Safewords are words or physical cues that can come up in the case of an emergency or need to pause the play. For example, three rhythmic grunts can show the need to check in for a Model who is gagged, or the military-themed scene can be paused with the words "Sir, no Sir." Some folks choose something even more deliberate, like the word "asparagus" meaning that either the Bottom or Top is finished, or using "red" for stop, "yellow" for pause and green for "go." Others choose a physical cue, such as dropping a bandana or jingly toy if the bound partner needs to pause the action or get untied.

Safewords do not have to mean "stop right now or I will sue you." The code you create may mean, "I have five minutes left," or "can we talk out of character?" No matter what system you create, make sure everyone is on the same page before your scene begins. It can be upsetting having one person think the word "gorilla" means "can we pause for a moment," and the other one thinks it means "get me out of rope now!" It may also be potentially damaging to a relationship or your partner's health.

For that reason, I encourage working with as clear of communication as possible when initially exploring together rather than relying on codes. "Ouch" means ouch. "Stop" means stop what you are doing. "Get me out" means please get me safely out of this tie. Ask questions in both directions to get further information, such as:

- Does that hurt?
- Is it a good pain, or a bad pain?
- How soon are we changing poses?
- Can you make this pose more challenging for me?
- Is this tie meant to be painful?
- How could we make this even hotter for you?

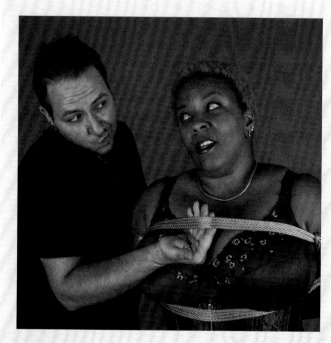

It seems a little loose.

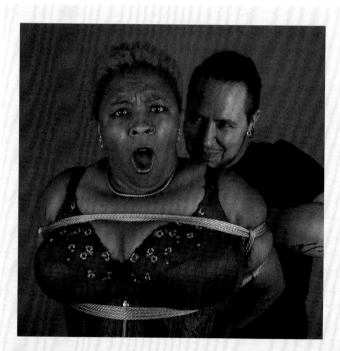

That is way too tight!

Sometimes a request to stop may mean your partner needs to change positions, or it may mean the entire scene is over. Finding out which desire a partner is trying to express, without judgment, can help immensely. The bulk of in-scene communication is not about safewords. By watching their face, their subtle shifts in body language and auditory responses (such as words, moans, and grunts), we build rapport with them. Being attentive and aware of their reactions can also help us be more present in the moment.

Tops, this does not negate your responsibility. Clear communication and safety are an active dance between partners. Checking in with your partner, avoiding body zones that you know are potential health risks, and staying alert and aware during a scene or erotic encounter can help keep you and your partner safe. Restraint may look simple and sexy, but simple issues can become big ones, so stay alert. Staying attentive and attuned with your partner also gives you a chance to connect on a deeper emotional level.

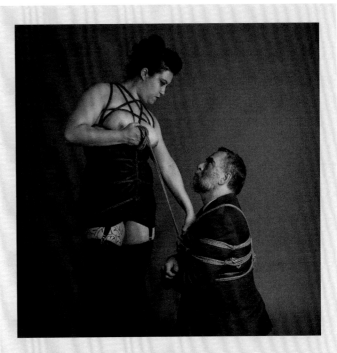

Be aware of what headspace someone is in when you negotiate. Not everyone can give full consent from a place of emotional submission.

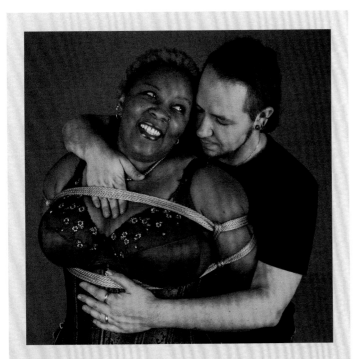

That is *just* right.

We can also choose to ask verbal questions of our playmate. They will have a chance to share their thoughts, feelings, and body experiences with us. It is also worthwhile to develop cues for keeping it all positive, rather than only sharing information when things are no longer good.

Be careful though. Some bondage Models think they need to tough out a tie, even if they are in horrible pain or have had a limb go numb. Others are in such an altered state of consciousness from the bondage that they don't realize how much duress their body is under. It is also possible for someone who is bound to forget how to communicate verbally. If you are a Bottom who toughs it out or knows they go into an altered state of consciousness (sometimes referred to as "sub space" or "rope space"), it is useful to share that fact before playing. Every Top will have to decide for themselves whether they feel comfortable tying someone who is no longer able to verbally communicate based on what they know about their partner.

Body Realities

Though we can bind chairs, guitars, or wine bottles, erotic rope bondage is intended to be done on human bodies. Whether we are decorating our own form, binding our lover, or doing performance art with friends, an awareness of our own body is key.

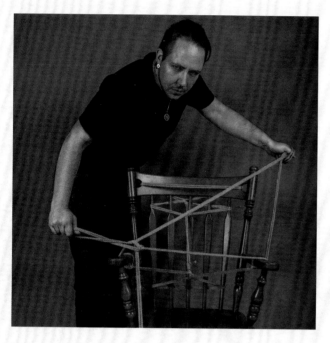

I guess we could tie up something other than a person...

We live in a world where we are taught to ignore our bodies. We work long hours on our feet or in uncomfortable chairs, and are told to "deal with it." However, when we are aware of pain, it becomes information we can use to reduce future pain in our lives. When we are aware of pleasure, it becomes information we can use to bring even more pleasure into our lives. We are able to share what gives us pleasure, and what to do to reduce the things that get in the way of that pleasure.

Sharing information with our lover about our joint challenges, past injuries or a troubled spine will reduce the chance of those things being an unexpected issue or disruption during a scene. Do you have allergies, asthma, or diabetes? Are you on any medications? Do you wear glasses, contacts, hearing aids, or prosthetics? Are you receiving ongoing mental health treatment or do you have phobias that might affect a bondage scene? Sharing these details in advance can help smooth things along, rather than finding out in the middle of a rope mummification that a Bottom is claustrophobic.

Tops, Riggers, and rope artists, this is important for you, too! Letting a partner know you have blood sugar challenges lets them know that getting you a snack pre-scene and post-scene will help your play be as fantastic as possible.

However, once we hear about body challenges, there may be a concern that the two of us are incapable of playing all together at all. This is not true. Trust and connection means that upon being vulnerable (about our fantasies or our body experiences) our partner will work with us to find solutions. For example we could have someone with a shoulder injury be bound asymmetrically and able to stay in rope longer, rather than being bound symmetrically and having to end the scene prematurely (or injure themselves).

The author, however, is not a medical professional. It is importance to do due diligence when making these decisions around your own body realities.

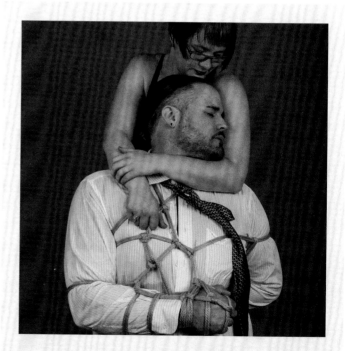

A shoulder injury can become an opportunity for artful and practical bondage.

Exercise: Learning Breath

Breathing and bondage are intimately interlaced. This applies not only to where on the body we tie, but how tight we tie and the positions we are contorted into. You can do the following exercise with yourself, or paired up with your play partner.

Sometimes having someone else assist will give us a less biased experience. There are times when we have a self-perception of how we breathe and move that may or may not match how we actually breathe and move.

Doing body-awareness exercises with someone else can help develop connection and trust. Other examples include watching our partner do slow stretching and giving feedback on what we see. If they moved with less flexibility on the left than on the right, we can share what we saw and learn if there are ties that would be better for their body. When sharing information with a partner about their body, try to do so with loving kindness.

No rope is needed for this exercise.

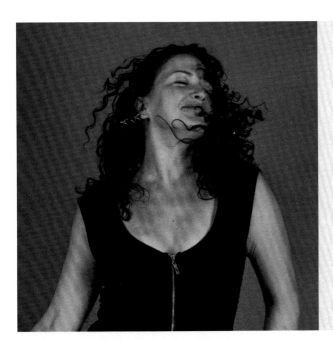

Loosen up

Shake out your body and relax your form. This is especially important after a long day of work. Consider slow stretching as well.

1

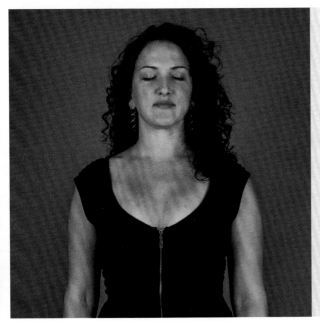

Breathe and relax

As you release the tension from your body, continue breathing normally.

2

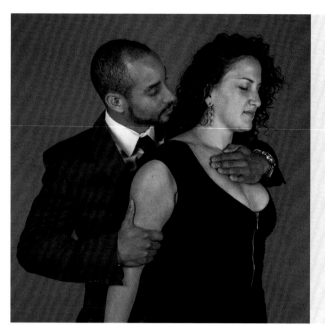

Upper chest

Have your partner place their hand on your upper chest. They should be able to notice how much it rises and falls as you continue to breathe normally for 30 seconds or more. Many of us lockup in exercises like this and do not breathe as we normally might. A normal breathing pattern is important.

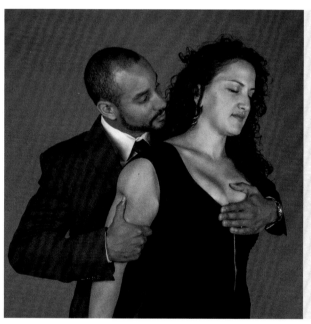

Mid-chest

Have your partner place their hand on your mid-chest. They should be able to notice how much it rises and falls as you continue to breathe normally.

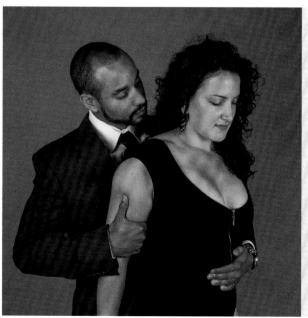

Diaphragm/belly

Have your partner place their hand just below your rib cage, at your diaphragm. They should be able to notice how much it rises and falls as you continue to breathe normally.

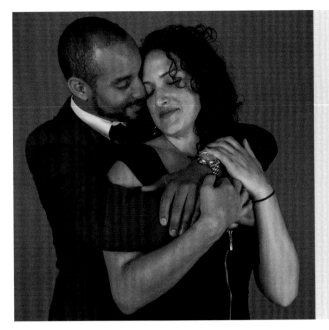

Compare notes

Thank or acknowledge your partner, and share what you noticed regarding where they breathed deepest. Process your findings.

6

This exercise is important because of the potential for positional asphyxia, which is the technical term for reduced airflow due to the pose we are in. It can be caused by cutting off the ability to get a full breath of air into the body, or by compressing the lungs, diaphragm, or rib cage in such a way that there is no way to take a breath.

Anyone can have this happen, and it is one of the many reasons autoerotic restraint (tying yourself up in a way that restricts movement for sexual pleasure) can be dangerous. This is doubly true when done alone, as no one is there to notice if your bondage has left you too

lightheaded to get yourself out of the tie. Assessing what type of "breather" someone is can help us reduce (but never fully eliminate) the chance of positional asphyxia.

Riggers—keep your own breathing style in mind as well. Are you a belly breather yourself? Instead of bending in half when tying your partner on the ground, consider sitting down next to them. Mid-chest breather? Wear a looser fitting top when binding lest you end up becoming light-headed.

Upper chest breathers have a greater chance of breathing issues with ties such as a chest harness if the upper chest rope is snugged tight. They may also have problems with ties where the upper chest has compression, is lower than the mid-chest, back-bends, or in poses where the upper chest gets constrained.

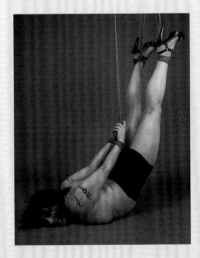

Chest down, ankles up

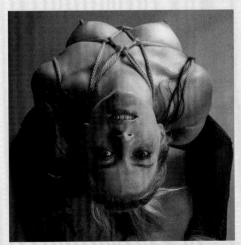

Tight chest harness or back bends

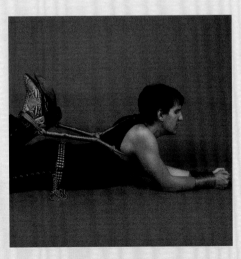

Upper chest ropes pulled back to ankles

Mid-chest breathers have challenges with ties that constrain the movement of the rib cage and upper/mid torso. This can include over-bust corsets, hog-ties, lashing to upright poles, or tight chest harnesses with extra pressure on the lower ropes.

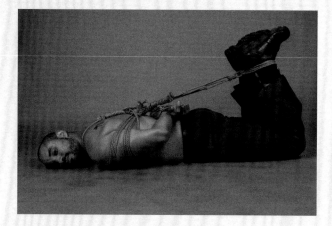

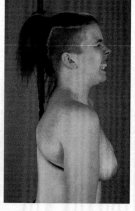

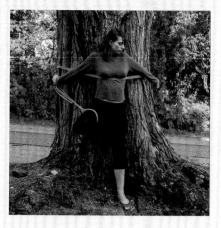

Gyaku Ebi (Asian-style Hogtie)

Attached to overhead point

Lashed tight under the chest

Belly breathers can have issues with ties that fold them in half, or put the full weight of their body on their midsection.

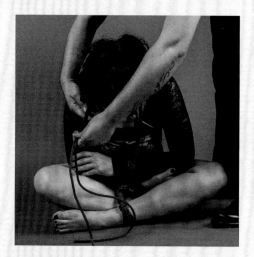

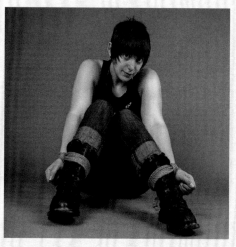

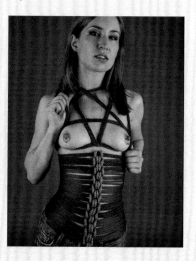

Ball Tie

Wrists to ankle, folded in half

Rope Corset

Just because your body breathes in a certain way does not mean you cannot do that pose! For example, if a belly breather is going to be hogtied, consider rolling them on their side from time to time, or propping their chest up with pillows. Don't aggravate the pose with challenging gags. Work with them to focus on slow, full breaths where each breath moves their upper chest.

Awareness of how we breathe can help us be bound for longer, and have it be a more enjoyable experience in the tie. Respecting our partner's limits is key. If someone says they can't breathe, it is better to err on the side of caution and change their position. Telling someone to "just breathe through it" is not always the appropriate choice.

Circulation and Nerves

When you tighten ropes at various points on the body, you can cut off blood supply. This leads to limbs changing color, tingling, losing the ability to grip, going cold, and eventually losing sensation.

A test for circulation begins by squeezing your Bottom's hand before you begin tying. Have them squeeze back, and encourage them to squeeze your hand or speak up if any challenges arise. Tell them that any time you squeeze their hand, you want them to squeeze back. Periodically, when the Bottom is tied, check their circulation in this manner. If their hand was warm at the beginning but now it's ice cold, can they still squeeze you firmly? If they can't open and shut their hand at all, it is time to move that limb. Are they squeezing back multiple times in rapid succession? They are likely trying to get your attention, and it is time to check in with them.

If you have to move a limb, is the scene over? Not if you don't want it to be! There are Models who get upset if they feel it is their fault they couldn't hold a pose. To offset negative emotions, consider saying something like, "I have an idea. I want to tie you this way instead." As a Rigger, you can claim the power to change poses. Make it your idea to move your partner, and affirm that having them share their experience is valued. This is also a chance to connect with them, touch their body, breathe with them, or add other intentions into your interaction. This is the case whether you are changing their pose, or giving them a quick break from having their wrists tied.

The other issue that can arise from rope bondage is nerve pain or impingement. If the bound person feels any unusual sensations including, but not limited to, electric shock running down their limbs, tingling, burning feelings, loss of sensation in half of the hand, pain, or weakness in the hand—act upon it. Move the limb or change the rope position as soon as you can without panicking. Nerve pain, if it continues, can lead to long-term or even permanent damage. Both extended duration circulation loss and nerve damage can cause serious problems.

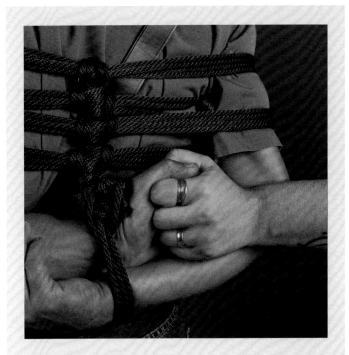

A squeeze can be a quick opportunity to check in.

Bottoms, speak up! If any of these issues arise, tell your partner. This is not the time to push through a tie, lest you risk your health and well-being. The likelihood of nerve and circulation impingement can be reduced by avoiding ties over the major nerves, arteries, and veins, and in various ties we will look at places to avoid pressure to some of these regions. Poses that involve hands being overhead challenge circulation as well, and hands in general can loose circulation. This is one of the reason to tie wrists last, or have speed-release options on ties that hold hands in place.

Unfortunately, not all nerve damage will manifest in obvious manners during tying. If after a scene circulation is overly slow to return, you have sudden pains of any sort caused by the rope or position, continued tingling or numbness persists, or a limb that is not responding as expected, don't be afraid to see a doctor. Most medical professionals are more concerned about getting you healthy than they are about your sexual preferences and predilections.

Flexibility and Stretching

Let's face it, very few of us are super-flexible fetish models. And that is ok—variety is the spice of life! Some individuals with extreme flexibility actually have other issues themselves, such as joints that slip out of socket or painful body tension.

It is perfectly dandy not to have your elbows, or even your wrists, touch behind your back. As you explore ties throughout the rest of this book, be honest with yourself. Some ties will come more easily, and others may need to be modified to your form. Consider using props such as chairs, pillows or beds to make a tie more doable.

Talk with your partner as you try out a pose. Let them know if your wrist hurts, shoulder pinches, back tweaks, or knees are uncomfortable. Turning that wrist, adjusting your shoulder position, or taking a few minutes to do some yoga in advance might help. Throwing a pillow under those knees can also help get them off a hard floor. Don't assume that because of someone's build that you know what poses they will be able to hold. There are small-framed people who can't have their hands behind their back, and people with a broader form who have high mobility.

Rope bondage can put your body through its paces. When running, it is usually encouraged to stretch out your body ahead of time, do a cool-down afterwards, and make sure to stay hydrated. Successful bondage incorporates all of these elements as well. Going for a run without warm-up can lead to a pulled muscle, and so it is for getting tied up or even being the Rigger! And just like not all runners can do a 10 mile run, if your body doesn't hold a certain pose, don't try to push your body into doing it.

Stretching comes in many different forms. It might be sports stretching, yoga, or hitting the dance floor. Perhaps you and your partner want to writhe around on the bed for a bit first, loosening up those tight muscles after a long day. It may surprise you how many core body muscles get engaged in a variety of these ties, whether you are the Model or the Rigger. Make sure to stretch not only in the direction that your body might be in a tie, but in the opposite direction as well. For example, if your arms will be pulled back, make sure to stretch them forward too.

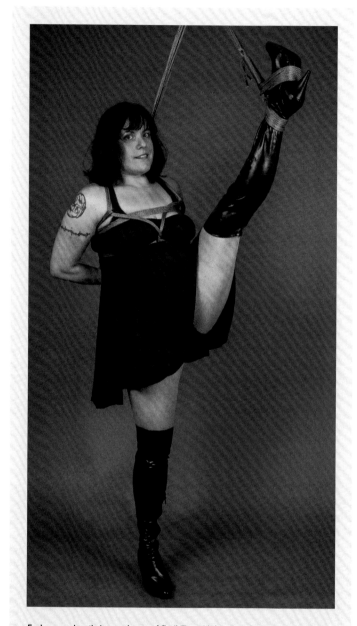

Each person has their own degree of flexibility, with honesty of experience being key.

Care for your body in general to have fun with bondage on both sides of the rope. Stay well hydrated to help your body stay limber. Consider some protein-based snacks, not just sugars, before and after you play. Keep options for warmth available in case your temperature drops. Have an eye on your own body needs, and watch out for one another. All of these will help you be more present energetically to one another, and lead to deeper emotional connections.

With all of these tools in mind... it is time to bind!

Columns and Cuffs

One of the basic ingredients for many bondage ties, no matter the position, is the cuff. A cuff is any item that wraps around a column of the body and is used to restrain or manipulate that body part. There are so many columns to choose from!

- Wrist
- Ankle
- Thigh (being careful with the femoral and sciatic nerves)
- Upper arm (being careful with the median, radial and ulnar nerves)
- Below the knee
- Waist
- Forehead (but not too tight)
- Center of the foot
- Cock and balls
- Size D+ breasts
- Neck (loose and pulling forward only, since pulling back or to the side is a choking hazard)
- Columns on a second (or third) person

The great thing about cuffs is that you can also tie columns other than those found on the human body:

- Tree trunks
- Pieces of furniture
- Bamboo poles
- and the ideas go on

However, not every part of the human body is a good candidate for a cuff to be tied around it. Some of these inappropriate location include:

- Front of the neck
- Inside or outside of joints
- Compressing or struggling on soft tissue
- Pressure on toes and fingers

Let's explore some ways to bind these various columns and learn to play around with this classic form of restraint.

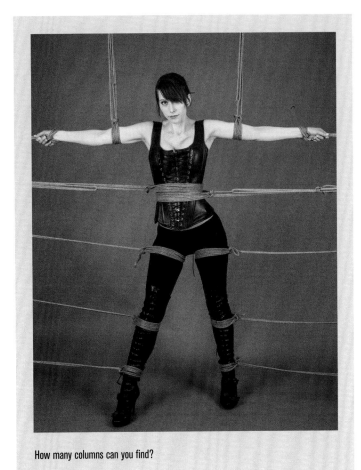

How many columns can you find?

Materials

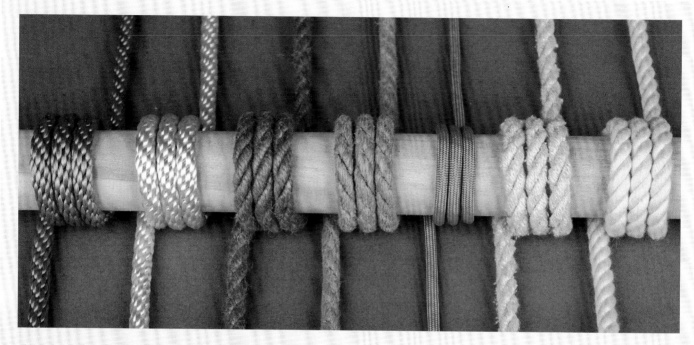

(From left to right) Multifilament Polypropylene (MFP), Nylon, Jute, Hemp, Paracord, Silk, Cotton

A cuff can be tied in a variety of materials. Artificial fibers (such as MFP, nylon and banda) are great because they are easily machine washable and less likely to expand when they get wet. Natural fibers with more texture/"tooth" (like jute and hemp) work well because they can hold knots easily and have a unique smell, which causes Pavlovian reactions in some rope Bottoms. Parachute cord is fantastic for detail work. Silk and bamboo are known as "luxury ropes" for their sensual caress. Flat webbing distributes pressure across a wider area. Cotton washes and holds a knot, but can become fluffy over time when washed and dried. Other options include climbing rope, marine line, leather lashing, polyester, and linen.

As for width, think about your interests and desires. If you want the ties to be more comfortable using distribution of pressure over a wider space, you might choose wider rope, or do more wraps around the column you are working on. If the bound partner is hoping for more challenging bondage, using rougher or thinner rope can provide that experience. Whichever route you choose, make sure to have your EMT shears or other emergency tools on hand for getting your partner out, just in case.

Various escape tools should be a part of every rope artists' kit. Have the device on your body or at the top of your toy bag so you can easily access it if needed.

Lengths of rope vary depend on what you want to do. Sometimes a long piece can seem like a good idea, but it can lead to tripping over your own rope. Remember you can always add on more rope (see page 50). If you are tying a **Somerville Cuff** (see page 26) around someone's wrist, and then attaching it to a bed or chair, a 10-15ft (3-4 meter) length is just fine. For a **Pentacle Harness** (see page 100), a piece or two that are 25-30ft (8-10 meter) in length may be in order. I prefer to have extra rope on hand, of different lengths, materials and colors, so I have just the right option for that moment. It can break the connection with my partners (and be unsafe) leave where we are playing to go get the supplies I forgot.

Choose for yourself what material you want to use based on the following questions:

- How much strain will there be on the line?
- How sensual do you want the texture to be?
- How many times will the line wrap around the body?
- Does color matter to you?
- Do you and your partners have any allergies to natural fibers, laundry soaps, or finishing oils?
- What smells turn you on?
- What is your budget?

Ask everyone involved these questions. Ideally, it is best to test out a variety of materials before investing a large amount of money in a type of rope just because a book or website told you to. No, really! If that polyester sash cord from the fabric store turns you on, have fun with it as long as you are doing decorative or bedroom bondage.

Ask everyone involved these questions. This especially matters before you invest in large volumes of rope. There are some amazing varieties of rope available on the market right now (see page 123), but buying 300ft (100 meters) of jute or hand-dyed polyester can be quite the investment. Consider going to events where you can feel the line in your hands (see page 124), or ordering sample pieces before you make a decision. Remember that you don't have to buy any specific type of rope just because a book or website told you to. If that polyester sash cord from the fabric store turns you on, have fun with it as long as you are doing decorative or bedroom bondage.

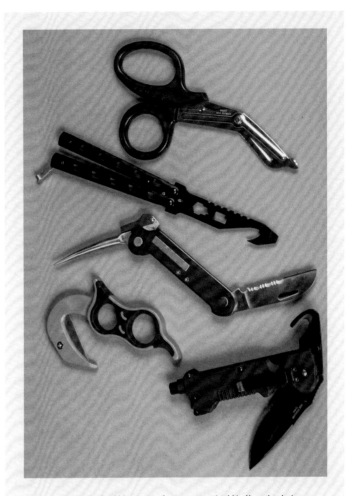

Various escape tools should be a part of every rope artists' kit. Have the device on your body or at the top of your toy bag so you can easily access it if needed.

Somerville Cuff

The Somerville Bowline was created by a Rigger named Topologist to address the issue of bondage situations under duress. The knots on the **One-Column Tie** (*Shibari You Can Use*) sometimes capsize, especially with artificial-fiber ropes such as MFP or nylon, making this bowline a superior tie for situations where the loops on that tie are not being used to catch or tie off.

With practice, this tie can become a very fast and efficient way to restrain someone, or a very sensual tie when done with confidence. Consider practicing in advance on your own ankle or a pole to get used to the way your hands move with the tie, building up muscle memory. Doing the rigging to a specific rhythm also allows you to speed up and slow down your tying once you have the specific tie memorized. Try turning the practice limb/pole upright as well as horizontal. It will give you expertise tying no matter which direction their body is twisted and turned.

Continued practice may lead to the ability to tie without looking at the ropes, enabling eye contact with your partner while laying ropes on them. This also builds confidence in your skills which will carry through to your partner. If you feel more comfortable, they will relax and feel more comfortable as well.

The tie here is shown using a 10-15ft (3-5 meter) length of 6mm jute rope for practicing the tie.

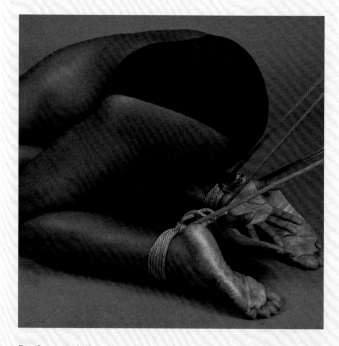

Four Somerville Cuffs can be used to create seemingly complex poses.

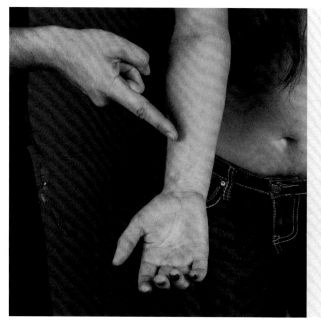

Find a column

Choose a column to bind. Identify anything you need to avoid, such as joints or the front of a neck. Ask in advance if the column might have other challenges, such as a wrist with a history of trauma. Covering a column with clothing can help make a tie more comfortable (and help avoid marks), and if your partner chooses to have their previously injured column bound, a brace may reduce the chance of further damage.

1

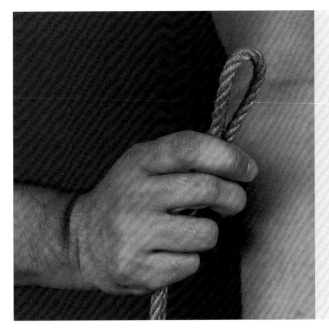

Make a bight

Fold your rope in half, creating a doubled line. The point at the middle of the rope is known as the "bight." Make sure there are no knots or debris in the rope. Feel the rope for splinters and see what the rope's burn speed is (how fast you can pull it without it hurting). This is a great opportunity to make eye contact with your partner, press up against their body, or pull the rope across their flesh as you fold the rope.

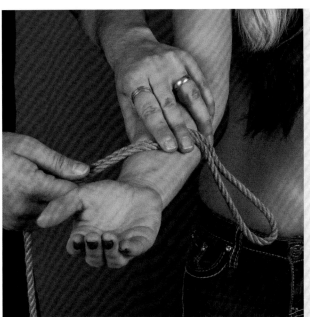

Place rope on wrist

Measure 5-10 inches (13-23 cm) from the bight of the rope (depending on how long you will want the tail/loop to be), placing a finger from your non-dominant hand over this starting point. This finger allows for the cuff to stay a bit loose, reducing the chance of wrapping too tightly.

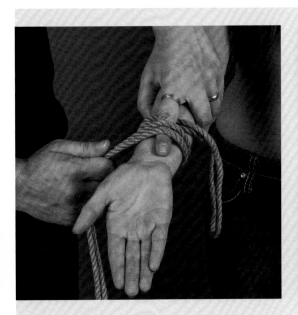

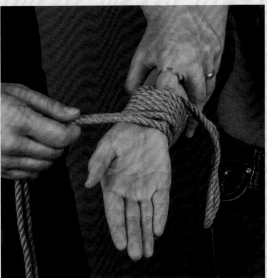

Wrap around the column three times

Wrap the long ends of the rope closer and closer to the wrist, going over the finger each time. Make sure there are no crossed ropes so pressure is distributed evenly.

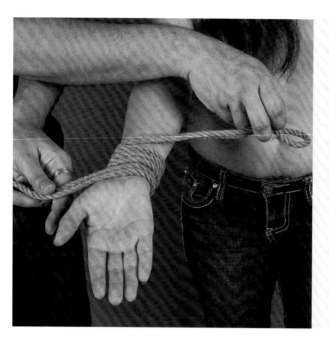

Remove spacer finger

Having wrapped three times around the column, remove the finger that was holding the space under the cuff.

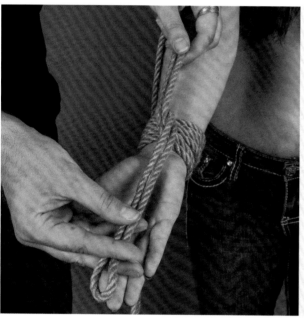

Twist or trade sides

In a wrist tie, since the bight end was nearest their elbow, it will now be pointing towards their fingers.

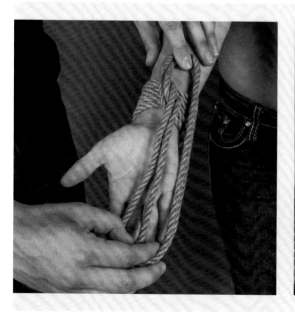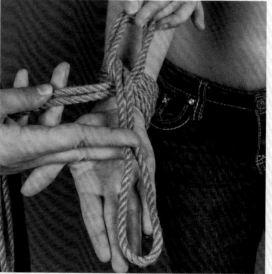

Create a loop

Using the long end of the rope, fold the rope back to create the letter "U," with the long end running over all of the wrist wraps. Then lift the short end of the rope slightly and lay the long end of the rope under the short end of the rope.

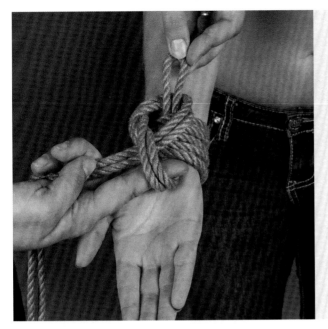

Pull bight under wraps

One option for this step is to insert a finger into the loop of rope nearest the elbow, then under the wraps, grabbing the bight of the rope and pulling it through. The other is to push the bight under all of the column wraps, coming out through the loop near the elbow.

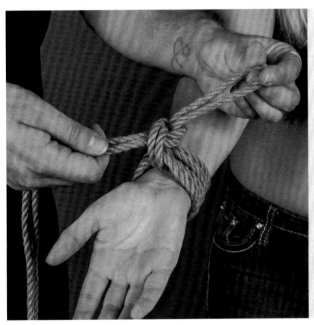

Tighten down the rope

Use both ends of the rope as you tighten down.

The finished **Somerville Cuff** is able to be pulled in any direction without the knot capsizing. It is practical for a wide variety of applications including:

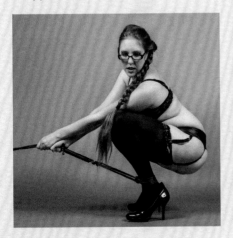

Ankle cuffs

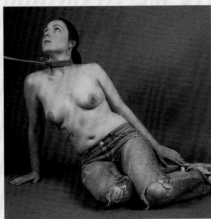

Collars

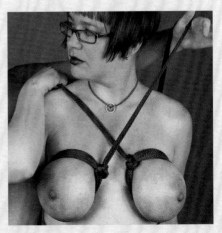

Large breast bondage

Pulley System

So how do you attach a wrist cuff, ankle cuff, or other cuff to a bedframe? What about a chair, table, or some other sturdy stationary object? Perhaps their chest harness? The following **Pulley System** is a way good to hold your partner in place.

Take a moment to consider if what they are tied to can take the strain. For example, the above ideas may be good, but don't tie them to sprinkler heads, curtain rods, luggage trolleys, or fresh genital piercings. Ouch!

Attaching to overhead points also carries a degree of risk if your partner becomes unconscious for any reason. Plan in advance, and have your safety tools for cutting rope (see page 79) easily accessible.

This book is for sensual, decorative, floor and bedroom-based bondage only. The issues of safety for suspension is not addressed in this book. Don't risk your partner's safety by using inappropriate equipment or ties for suspension.

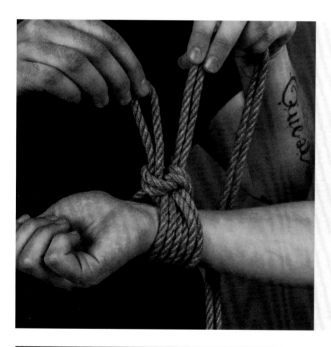

Find the running end and the bight

When using the **One-** or **Two-Column Tie** from *Shibari You Can Use* or the **Somerville Cuff** (see page 26), there are two available sets of ends when the tie is finished. The little loop is not a design flaw—it is a design feature!

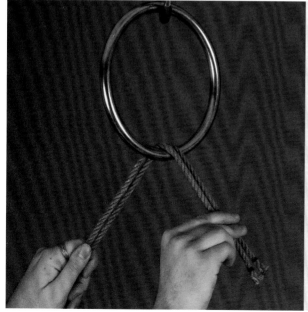

Go around/through attachment point

Take the running end of the rope, and wrap around the attachment point, or pull through it, depending on what you are attaching to.

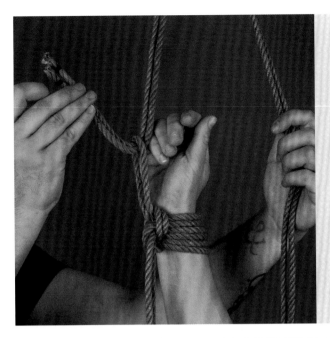

Pull running end through bight

Come back from your attachment point, and run the loose ends of the rope through the bight of the rope.

3

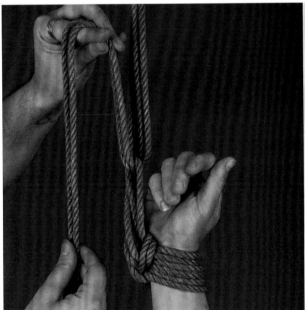

Adjust tension

Reverse tension on the line. This is done by going back the way you just came. Using a pulley helps you determine how tightly you want the bondage restricting your partner, and allows you to later loosen or tighten the bondage.

4

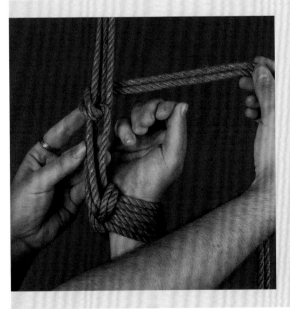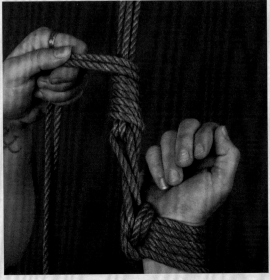

Wrap around all ropes

Pull together all the ropes just above your bight. Wrap around all of the lines a few times, with 3 wraps as a minimum. More can be beautiful, is fine, but the more you wrap, the more you have to unwrap later.

5

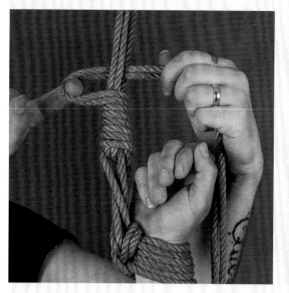
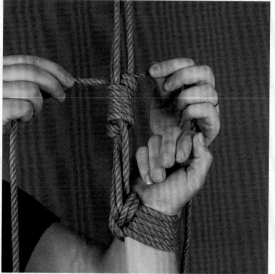

Tuck through

Split the four lines of the rope attached to your structure, with two lines on each side of the gap. Take the running ends of the rope and tuck them through before tightening down.

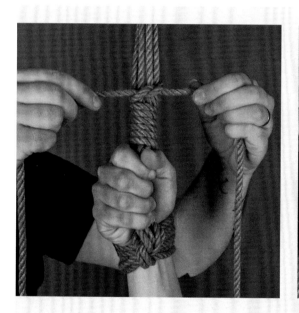
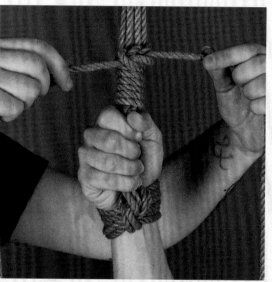

Tie off

Split the lines apart, and bring each line around in opposite directions. Tie a square knot where the lines meet on the opposite side. The tie is now secured and ready for your partner to pull on.

Slipped Pulley System

For some people, pulling the ends of the rope all of the way through can feel slow. This is especially the case when working with long ropes, or doing speed bondage. The finished Slipped Pulley System may not have the same aesthetics as the classic Pulley System, but is fast and efficient. Being efficient can provide more time to focus on our partner.

You may find that you and your partner enjoy one pulley more than another. For example, if you are playing with an "eel" (a Bottom who enjoys being an escape artist), doing the basic Slipped Pulley may be a poor fit, but experimenting with the optional steps at the end may help the tie be a success. If, on the other hand, the two of you enjoy quick transitions between rounds of relaxing into your rope, this system is for you.

Follow steps 1-5 from the **Pulley System** on page 30 (perhaps using fewer wraps for speeding up the tie) and change the last steps to the following:

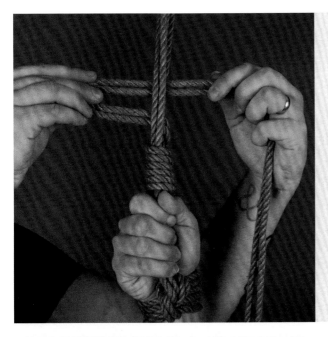

Fold the rope

Fold the rope a 3-4 inches (10 cm) from where the wrapping ends. This becomes a secondary "bight." Push the secondary bight through the gap created by pulling the four ropes apart. Do not pull the rope all the way through. Only pull through the secondary bight and a few extra inches.

6

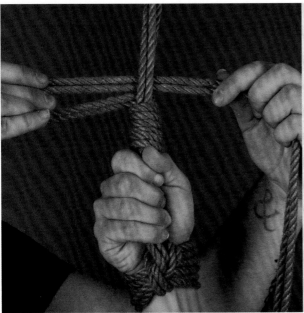

Push down

Push down to lock the tie. The quick-lock (held still by the friction between the split ropes and your partner pulling on the rope) is finished for short-term restraint.

7

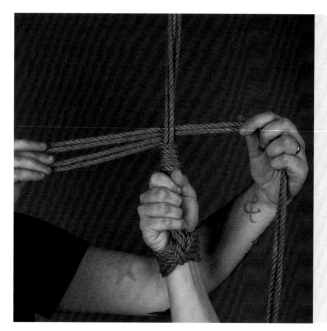

(optional) Extend secondary bight

If someone will be in a pose for more than a few minutes, or might squirm, you can more securely lock off the Slipped Pulley System. Begin by pulling the secondary bight a foot (30 cm) beyond the lines that were tucked through.

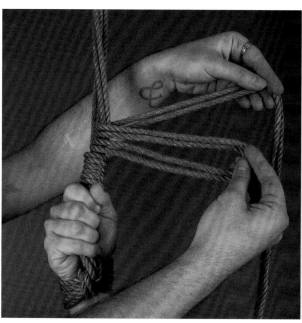

Fold rope

Fold the lines over so they all face the same direction.

Tie off

Tie a half hitch knot and tighten down. The completed tie can now be pulled upon and will not loosen, even when struggling.

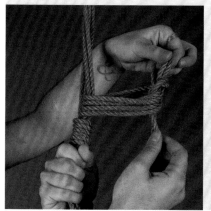
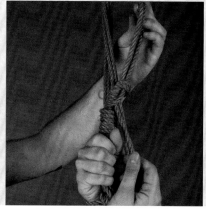
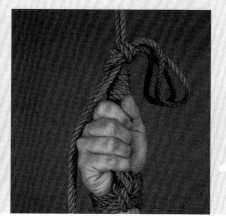

Changing Positions

The great thing about either pulley system is that if your partner starts having challenges with their hands, a scene does not have to stop. For example, hands can go tingly or fall asleep, perhaps indicating circulatory issues. Loosen the cuff by adjusting the pulley and tying off again. Changing the tension on the line usually addresses the concern.

If the pose no longer is meeting your desires, it can be modified to a different position without your play partner being completely untied. This can help maintain a sense of continuity within a scene or encounter, as compared to removing all of the rope from a partner's form and then retying from scratch. Changing positions can keep the play going.

You don't even have to wait for their hands to fall asleep to change it up—sometimes it's just fun! Moving from being bound face down (see page 26) to being spread-eagled on your bed can be great for sex play or a sensual experience using light touch.

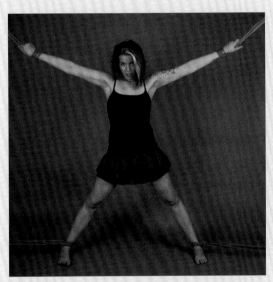
Perhaps you are done with this position

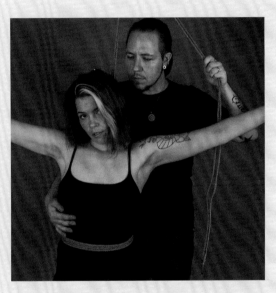
Add a support line at their waist

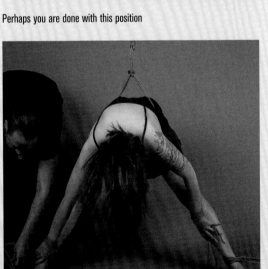
Maneuver them into the new position

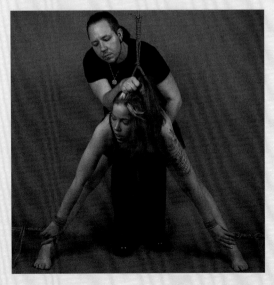
Tie off and enjoy!

Texas Handcuffs

Ever wished you had a pair of handcuffs, but only have a piece of rope? Wish that handcuffs were more comfortable to be in, or more pliable? Want a speed tie that you can slip on your partner? The Texas Handcuffs are right for you.

There a variety of versions of this tie, and the one shown here is two basic slip knots paired at the center. The more you practice between scenes, the quicker your can get due to it's simple form.

Because this tie is made of slip knots, make sure to pull your ropes in opposite direction when tightening down, rather than holding one rope still and wrapping around with the other rope. If you only pull on one side, your "prisoner" is certain to escape. Pulling down only on one side can also turn that side into a tourniquet, cutting off circulation on that side.

The tie here is shown using a 10-15ft (3-5 meter) length of 6mm MFP rope.

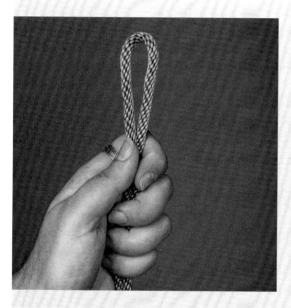 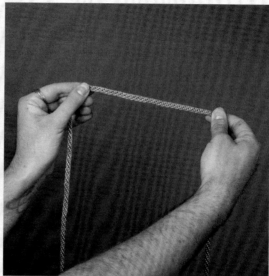

Find the middle of your rope

You are not creating a bight by keeping the rope folded. This is only done to find the middle, which is located in the second picture in the space between hands.

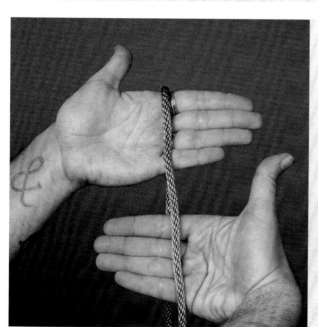

One hand left, one hand right

Rest the rope on top of your fingers, with one hand pointing to the left, and one hand pointing to the right, both with your palms facing up. Give yourself distance between your two hands, with the middle of the rope in the gap between those hands.

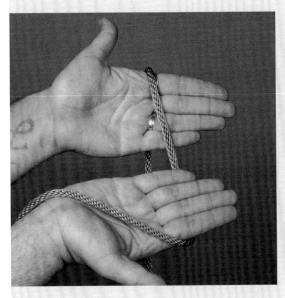
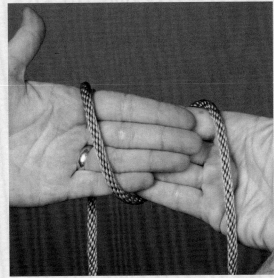

Tips of fingers together

Twist your right/lower hand clockwise, until your fingertips are pointed in the same direction. Now twist the right hand counterclockwise, sliding the right hand behind the left. Keep your fingers in contact, with no rope between your hands.

3

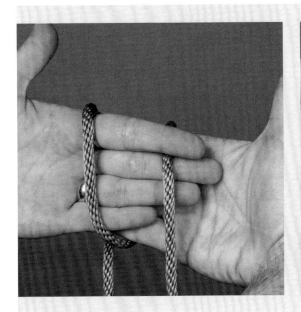
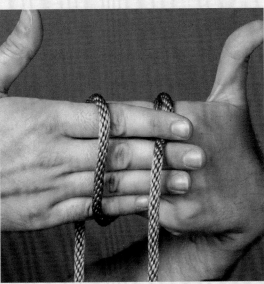

Grab the ropes

Using the space between your left index and middle fingers, grab the rope. Using the space between your right index and middle fingers, grab the rope.

4

Pull away

Pull your hands apart. Keep holding onto the part of the rope you grabbed between your fingers. Keep holding. Tighten up the knot.

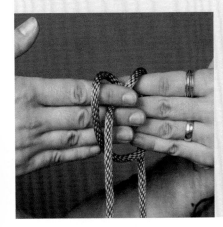
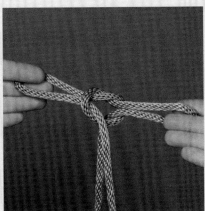
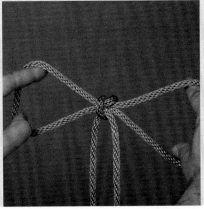

5

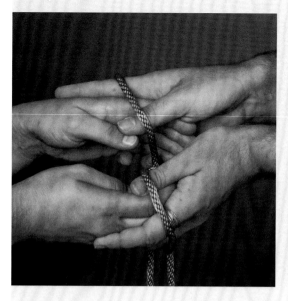
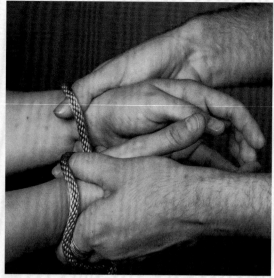

Slip columns into the loops

Put a hand through each loop. Your partner can slip their own hands through, or you can grab their hands (with the loops resting on your own knuckles).

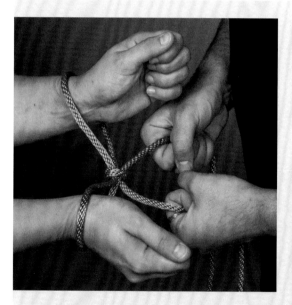
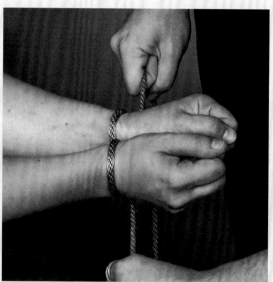

Tighten down loose ends

Grab a loose end in each hand, and pull your hands apart. Pull snug. Tighten down enough that they cannot escape, but not tight enough that you cause nerve damage or cut off circulation.

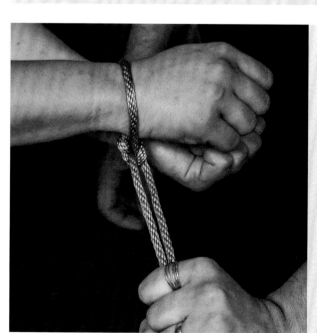

Bring ends together

To hold the tension in place, bring the loose ends together and keep tension on both lines.

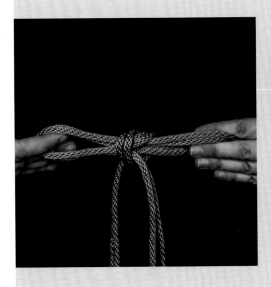 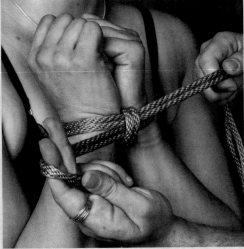

(optional)
Doubled line

If you want someone in this tie to be more comfortable, consider the issue of pressure distribution. If your rope is only 6mm wide, all of their struggling will be on that very small area. Ouch. If you use a rope that is twice as wide, it will be twice as comfortable. A folded rope (needing to start out at least twice as long) can help your Bottom stay bound longer.

9

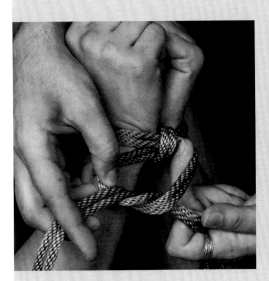 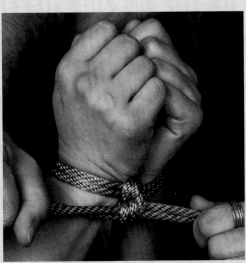

(optional)
Overhand knot

You will need to lock this pair of slip knots if you are going to release tension on the line. If your "prisoner" is trying to escape, pin their hands together during tying off. Additional overhand knots are advised for slippery ropes such as nylon, MFP, and polyester.

10

Exercise: A Whisper or a Kiss

The desirous touch. The needful whimper. For many of us, this is what bondage is about. Watching our partner's reactions. In this exercise, we will use the Texas Handcuffs to illicit a response from our partner.

Please adapt the following technique as appropriate to your relationship. For example, if you are not sensually or sexually intimate with your partner, you may want to pull their hands back and end the exercise there. For others, you may linger at the genitals, using the rope as a vibrator or point of tension as you move it back and forth. Knowing your partner and their "whys" can help you determine what is best for both of you and the moment.

Remember that the exact tie is not the focus of this exercise. If you are concerned about whether you know how to tie the knots, practice them in advance before trying out this combination experiment. If, during the exercise, you forget the tie, it's okay. What matters is connection and reaction, not the details, as long as you are not putting your partner at risk.

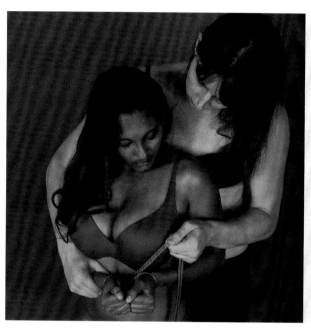

Texas Handcuffs

Stand in close proximity to your partner, whether in front or behind them. Tie a pair of **Texas Handcuffs** on your partner, with their wrists in front of their body. Lock it off with an overhand knot. Since their arms will be lifted up behind their head, the wrist bindings need to be left slightly loose as the tie will tighten when the elbows are forced apart.

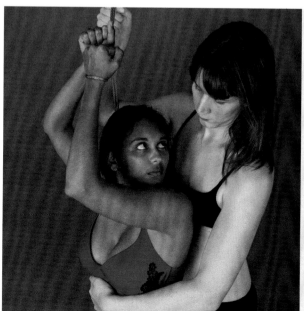

Arms overhead

Using the running end of the rope, slowly raise their hands over their head. Lean in close as you do so, wrapping your arm around their body, both to keep their balance and to increase physical contact.

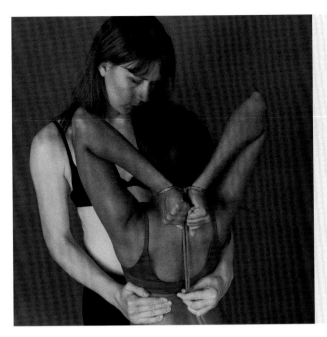

Arms behind

Bring their hands down, with their elbows pointed towards the sky. The rope is still in your hand, which is now pointed towards the ground. Don't let the rope leave your hand. Keeping tension on the rope reminds your partner that you are still present and with them, and can increase their sense a safety.

3

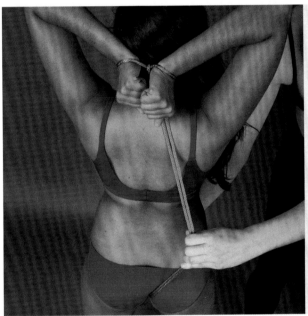

Between the legs

Run the rope up between their legs. Try using one hand to hold the rope in back, then reach through the legs to grab the rope using your other hand. If your partner is nude, this rope has become a crotch rope and needs to be washed between partners, or dedicated to this individual. You can run the rope up the middle, to one side, wrap it around external genitalia, or split the rope apart to frame each side of the pubic area.

4

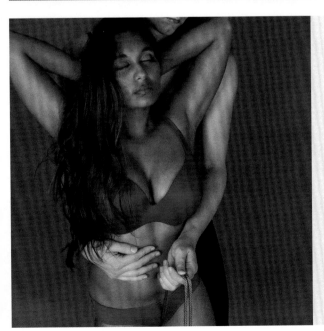

Bring the line up

Pull the rope up, and rest your other hand against their pubic mound, solar plexus, or heart. Each of these body zones can feel intimate in different ways, encouraging sexual response, security, or loving attachment. Maintain tension on the line.

5

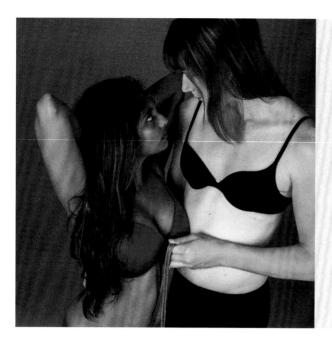

Breathe

Lock eyes with your partner. Watch how your Bottom is breathing and then match time with them. Breathe together.

Lean forward and either slowly kiss them, or whisper in their ear. For some this might evolve into a passionate lip-lock, while others might choose to breathe a growl for their partner to hear.

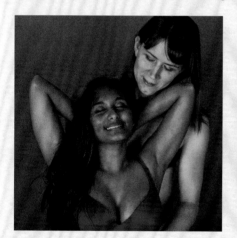

Will you smile or laugh with them?

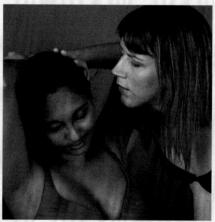

Whisper something sweet?

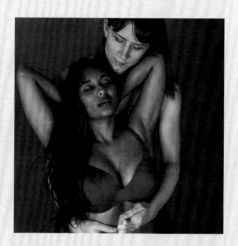

Or find yourselves in a passionate embrace?

Where are they emotionally and energetically today? Listen to what they verbally told you as well as what their body language is projecting. If in doubt, especially with a new partner or when trying something new, gently ask in a way that will not "break the spell" of your encounter. If what their body language is projecting is different then what has been negotiated, it is often best to stay within the negotiated lines and then debrief afterwards. After all, we want to connect with our partners... and get to play again later!

Doing otherwise is a form of "edge play" where there is risk involved. The risks in this case is that we might hurt our partner emotionally or physically, and affect how they see us. A Bottom is putting a great deal of trust in their Top, and deserves to have that trust held up. Everyone in kinky play deserves to have a partner who will respect us and our comfort levels. After all, we want to connect with our partners... and get to play again later!

Upper Body Ties

Whether we call them chest harnesses, torso constriction, boob bondage, pectoral decoration, or upper body ties, the concept is the same—putting rope on above the waist and below the neck. They can be done on a variety of body types, and can be great foundations for complex ties... or be delicious on their own!

Are you decorating someone for a party? Putting them in a challenging position? Perhaps your desire lies in objectification, or even erotic embarrassment. This examination in advance can help you design something perfect for your delight.

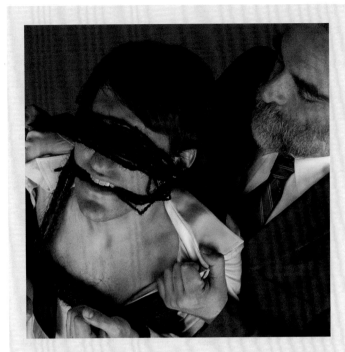

For a more sadistic approach, materials like horsehair, coconut, or unprocessed hemp can make for an intense experience. Keep those eyes closed!

Consider your materials. A chest harness made of colorful MFP or nylon (even multiple colors in one tie) can be visually dramatic. Jute and hemp look very classical for Asian aesthetic ties, and cotton can have a very "Western bondage" feel. Thin cord like parachute cord, or even dental floss, can be an extreme ordeal for upper body ties. Have those safety scissors nearby and be careful if you choose to bind over the upper arms that are full of nerve bundles. Lace can be a beautiful option, as can leather cording or yarn. Be creative; use what works best for the intent of your ties.

While you are being inventive, remember how your partner breathes (see page 17). A tight upper rope or tight lower rope will affect different Bottoms in a variety of ways. To affect their breathing, you can also choose to have them breathe out as you put on the ropes which will have the ropes feel very tight when they breathe in. The reverse can be done by tying when their lungs are full, leaving the harness loose later on. Be careful of escape artists though! They might puff up just to make their flight that much easier.

There are additional upper body ties in Chapter 6 that have been modified from the collection of chest harnesses shown in *Shibari You Can Use*. Those ties, along with the ties shown here, help show just how diverse and creative the opportunities for rope artistry can be.

Floral Harness

This decorative harness starts with a moderately complex knot called the **Floral Knot**, which is sometimes known as a five-petal Good Luck Knot. Spending the time to tie complex knots in advance can let your partner know that you were thinking about them before the scene ever began. However, if you are tying the knots during the scene, it can take time to construct. Consider connecting with your partner as you create it to make sure they do not get bored or feel disconnected from you. This can include having them curl up behind you, kissing them before you begin tying, or having them assist the scene by laying out other supplies.

There are a wide variety of decorative knots that can be added to your rope bondage that will make your rope bondage stand out as ties inspired by the world of macramé. For inspiration, check out some of the knot sites and books in Chapter 7. Though some artistic knots may not be appropriate for restraint, they may be perfect for crafting visually appealing ties. Even classic macramé books from the 70s can be fun to study for ideas of how to decoratively bind your lover.

This tie uses one 20-35ft (6-11 meter) piece of rope, depending on the frame of your partner.

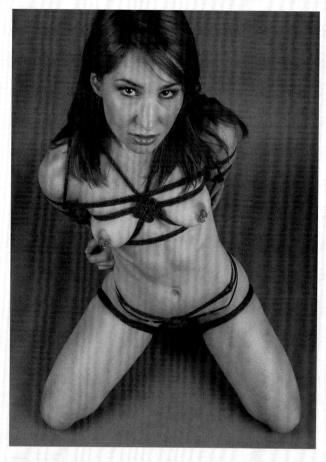

Floral Harness combined with a Box Tie (*Shibari You Can Use*), and Triskelion Crotch Rope (page 88).

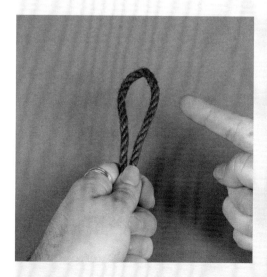

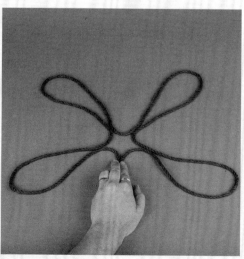

Create four petals

Find the middle of your rope. Lay the lines out on the ground, with the middle of the rope as the low point of the two central petals. Each of the "petals" of this Floral Knot will be about one foot long as we begin tying. Using your two loose ends as the fifth petal, lay the rope out into a star pattern, with each petal equally separated from each other.

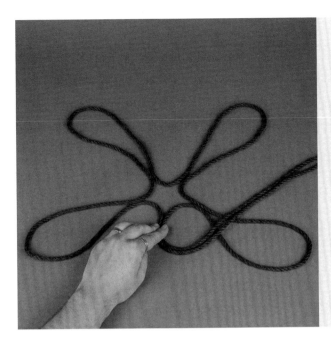

Lay lines counterclockwise

Beginning with the loose/long ends, lay the lines over the next petal/loop.

2

Repeat

Repeat step 2 with the next three petals, crossing over both the line that was just laid and the next petal.

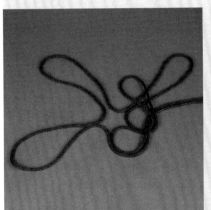 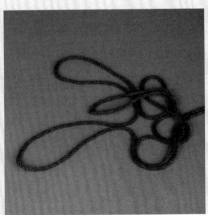 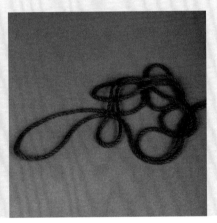

3

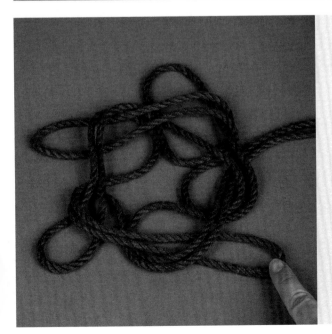

Lay and tuck under

Repeat the clockwise laying over with the fourth petal, crossing over the line that was just laid, then tucking underneath the one with the original loose/long ends. This will create a completed circle of ropes that look like a flower.

4

Tighten the lines

Snug down each rope a little bit, then tighten the next rope, and the next. This will help keep consistent tension on the ropes to create your star shape. Pulling on only one line will create a lopsided knot. If you find there are twists in your lines as you tighten, take the time to untwist them and make sure the knot lays flat.

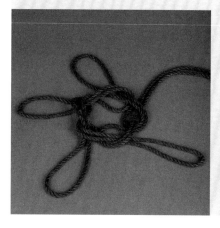 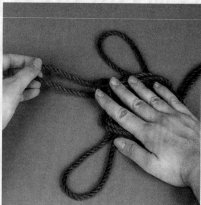 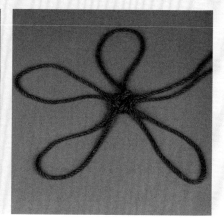

Reverse directions

Beginning with the loose ends, lay over the next petal, this time clock-wise. With each of the following petals, cross over both of the line that was just laid as well as the next petal.

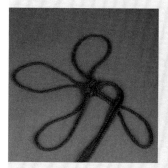 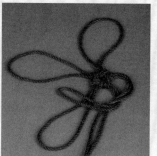 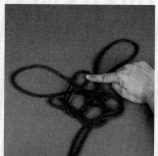 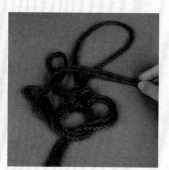

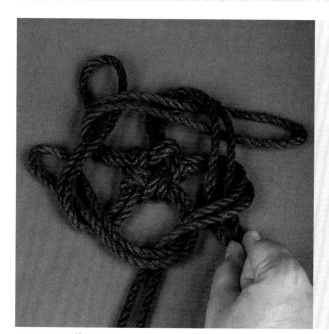

Lay and tuck under

Repeat the counterclockwise laying over with the last petal, crossing over the line that was just laid, then tucking underneath the first petal (the one with the loose ends). This will create a completed circle of ropes that looks like a flower. The hand in the image is keeping the knot steady, as sometimes the tips of ropes may slide around.

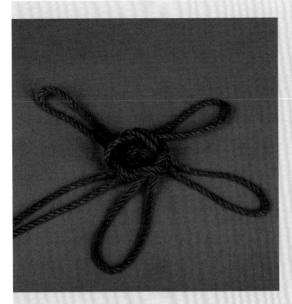
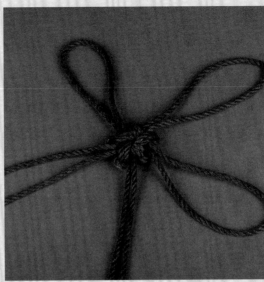

Tighten the lines

Snug down each petal a little bit, then tighten the next petal, and the next, as you did in **step 5**.

8

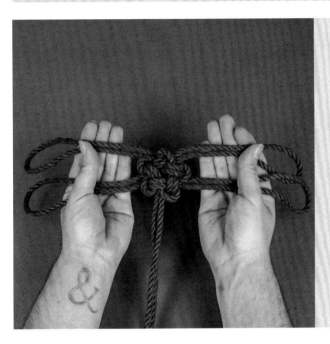

Flip over

You have now completed the large Floral Knot! Now let's get this onto our partner, shall we?

9

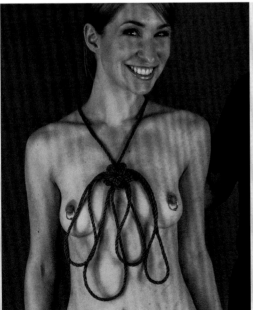

Center the knot

Place the knot directly over the sternum, with the loose ends at the "top" of the knot. You can have them hold the knot in place, which creates a great opportunity for collaborative creativity, or do it yourself with a firm hand, asserting dominance. Sometimes though, the person being bound is just giddy to be being decorated... even if the lengths of the petals aren't quite even.

10

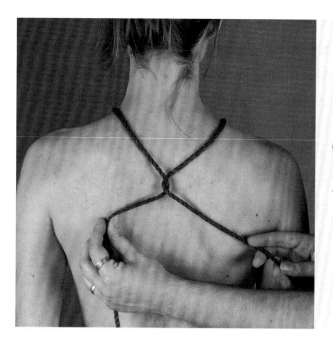

Over the shoulders and twist

Run the loose ends over each shoulder, and twist when you get to the back.

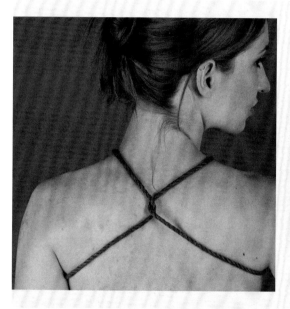

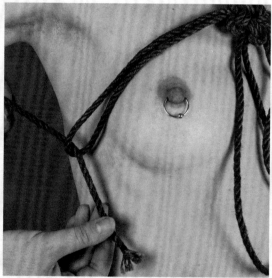

Run to the front and catch

Bring one loose end onto each side of the torso, and "catch" the top petals by running through them from bottom to top. The rope will lay above the breasts or pectoral mass.

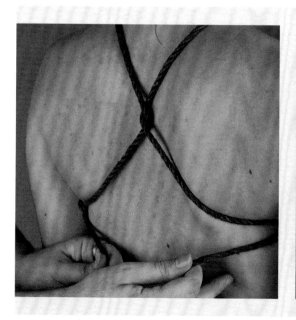

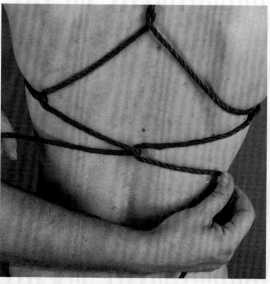

Bring to the back and twist

Snug the chest line down to create the firmness you want in the finished tie. Now bring the ropes to your partner's back, and twist.

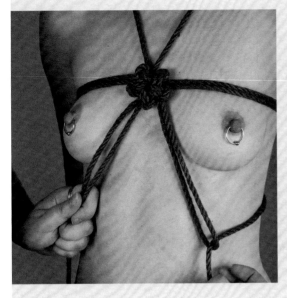
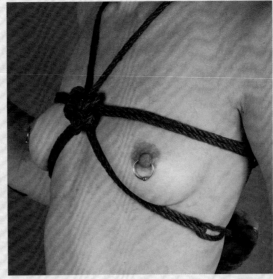

Run to the front and catch again

Bring a loose end onto each side of the torso, and "catch" the bottom petals by running through them from bottom to top. The rope will lay below the breasts or pectoral mass.

14

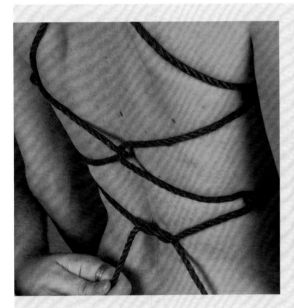
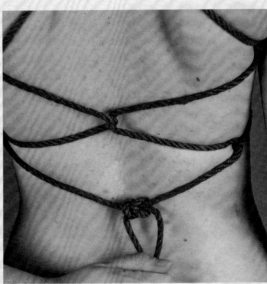

Bring to the back and tie off

Adjust the chest harness to create the snugness you want in the finished tie. Bring your ropes together and tie off with a square knot.

15

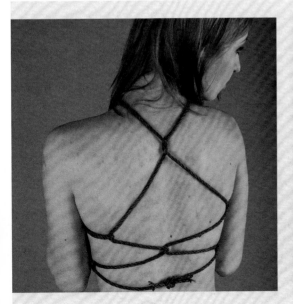
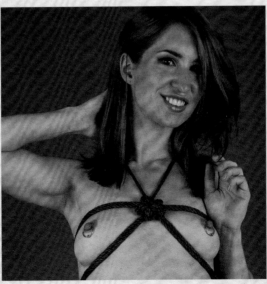

Bring to the back and tie off

Voilà! One finished Floral Harness!

16

Adding on Rope

Ever run out of rope and wanted to keep going? You are not alone—everyone does. By practicing this tie ahead of time, you will be ready when just such an issue arises. Knowing how to add rope creates an opportunity to use a number of 25-30ft (8-10 meter) pieces that are more easily manageable, rather than 50-60ft (17-20 meter) pieces that can be unwieldy.

The practice example here is shown in two different colors to enable easier following of the concepts. This is not to infer that different colors need to be used. Though it can be fun to use running out of rope as an opportunity to change colors or media, other folks prefer to use the same types of line throughout their rigging.

Two additional techniques for adding on rope are shown in *Shibari You Can Use*. What matters is that you know a technique, and can do it without having it distract from your scene. You can even use these moments as a chance to pull a lover in close for a kiss.

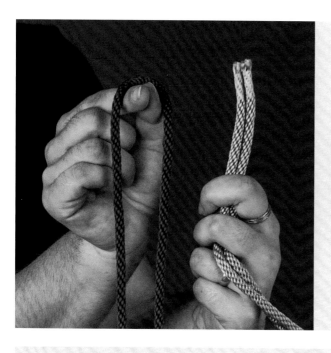

Find the bight

Find the bight of your new rope. Have the ends of your old rope either in your other hand, or easily accessible.

1

Create a lark's head

Spread the middle of the bight open using your thumb and forefinger while holding the line 6+ inches (15+ cm) down, forming a triangle. Flip the hand with the triangle over, creating a shape that looks vaguely like mouse ears. Put your thumb and forefinger together, and shake the line down onto itself. There you go! Lark's head.

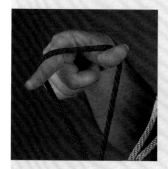 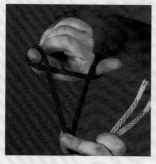 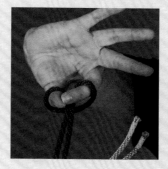 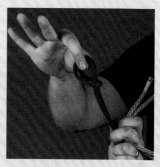

2

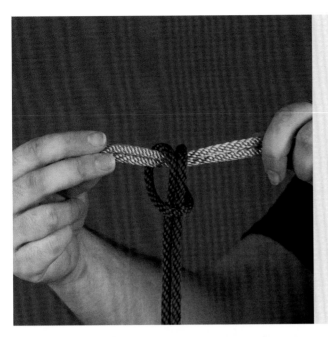

Slide lark's head onto old line

Take the two loose ends of the old rope, and slide the lark's head 3-6 inches (8-15 cm) up the line.

3

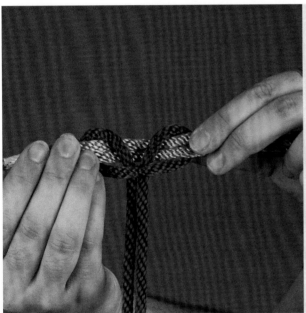

Open the lark's head up

Lay it flat along the line.

4

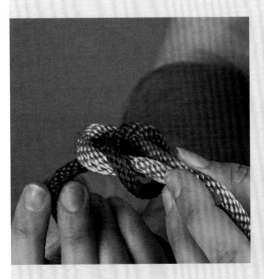

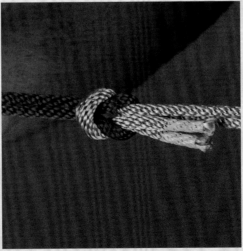

Fold the old rope

Take the two lines of the old rope and fold them back on themselves. The fold created in the old ropes will be at the center of where the lark's head has been split open.

You are now ready to start tying once more. If the knot will be in an uncomfortable place, you can have your fold be further up the line. The knot will lock in place wherever the fold is!

5

Reverse Box Tie

The Reverse Box Tie is a form of bondage which is fantastic for poses where our partner will be lying on their back, or when engaging in sexual play. It is also an option for those whose body is not suited for pulling their hands behind their back.

The step-by step version of this tie is shown using two 25-30ft (8-10 meter) pieces of MFP and one 15ft (5 meter) piece of MFP, but lengths of rope needed will vary depending on the Model being bound. MFP is being used to show where different ropes begin and end during instruction, but the finished ties are shown using one consistent material and color.

As this is a complex tie, remember to pause every once in a while. Look up from the bondage and catch the eye of the person you are binding. Take a moment for a smack on the ass, a hard hair pull or a sensual stroke if that sort of connection is desired.

Any time you need to add rope (see page 50), do so, making sure that the adding points are not in tender areas (such as the armpit) or areas where pressure will be placed on the tie when the box is completed (such as the outside of the arm if they will be lying on their side).

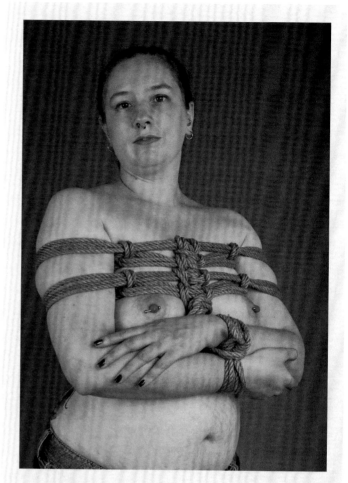

Reverse Box Tie

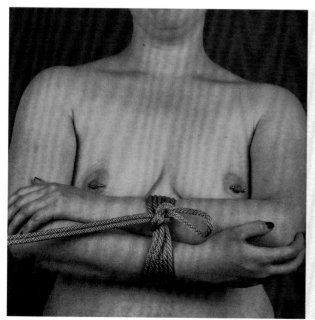

Tie cuff

Position the arms folded in front of the body, and bind the wrists together as if they were a single column. In this case, we used a **Somerville Cuff** (see page 26).

Transform into two columns

Run the long end between the wrist and forearm on one side, and have it come back to the front on the other. Having done so, tuck the long ends underneath the lines that began the transformation. A modification of this tie can be done by using a **Two-Column Tie.** (as shown in *Shibari You Can Use*)

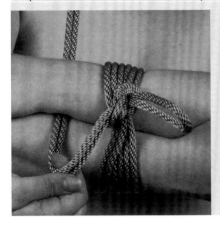 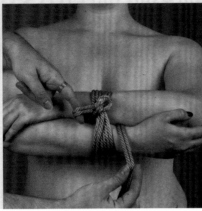 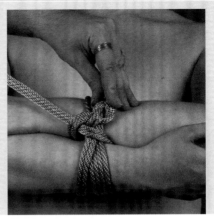

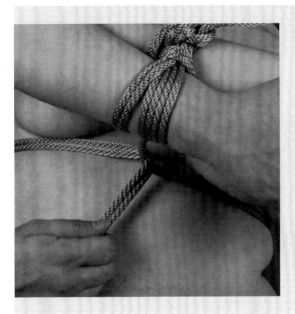 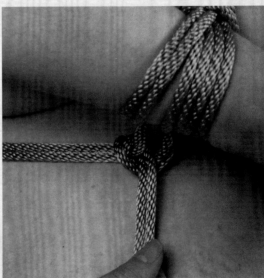

Attach to torso

Bring the line between the arms and downward behind the lower arm. From there, run the loose ends around the torso at wrist-height. Catch the line where it began, and tie off with an overhand knot.

Bring line up and wrap twice

Pull the line up behind the wrists, and angle up towards the right. Bind the body wrapping around the right shoulder and above the chest. Continue around the chest a second time, allowing the rope to cross over the line that runs from the wrist up to the first wrapping.

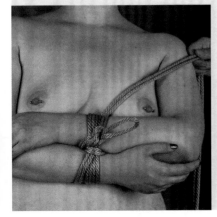 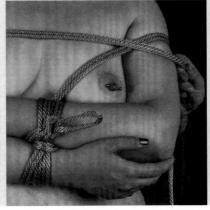 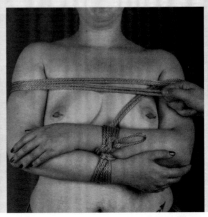

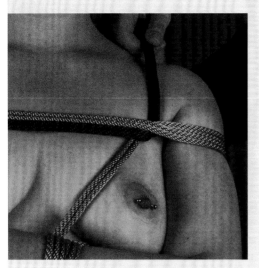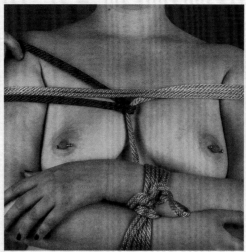

Catch the lines

As the second wrap comes back to the start of the upper chest wraps, hold the piece of rope you are working with on the outside of the wrapping lines, and pull the long end up underneath all of the upper chest wraps.

Having moved your rope underneath all of the upper chest lines, securely pull everything tight, pulling towards the center of the body.

Lock the stem

Start locking off the stem by bringing the rope in your hand down to the left. Slide the rope underneath the stem. Bring the rope back up over the chest wraps. Finally, bring it down behind the chest wraps, coming out on the left side of the stem.

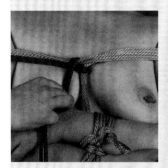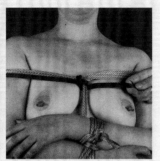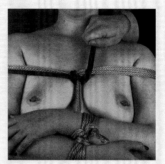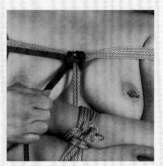

Secure the right upper wraps

Begin by bringing the rope through the open space on the right side of our Bottom's body between their armpit and elbow-pit. Once through, carefully bring the line up under the chest wraps, snugging up into the armpit while applying tension, but not hurting the sensitive tissue in that region.

Once the rope is in place, pull it down, and return to the front of the body going through the same open space you emerged from. Do not snug down too tightly, as cinching on the back side of the arm can cause pressure over nerve bundles near the surface of the skin.

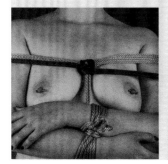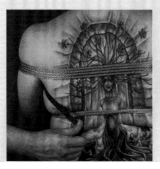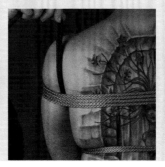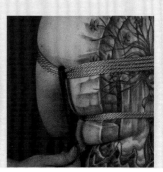

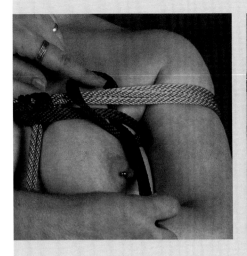

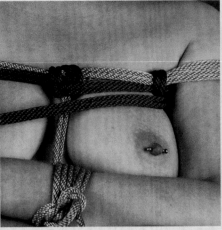

Hook the right upper chest wraps

Because people usually have more mobility moving their shoulders forward than they do moving them back, it is important to hook the front of the upper wraps before continuing on. Create an overhand knot that wraps around not only the initial four lines, but the two lines that were just laid when you secured the back of the right arm. Make sure the tie is snugged towards the armpit, but again, do not tighten down too tightly. Doing so can create a tourniquet around the arm. This hitch will stop the upper arms from being able to pull forward.

8

Secure and hook the left upper wraps

Crossing over the stem in the front of the body, **repeat steps 7 and 8** on the left hand side.

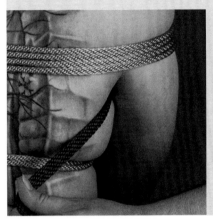

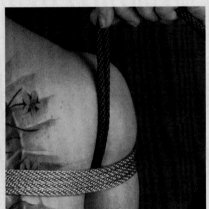

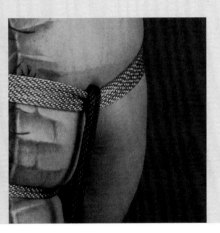

9

Lock the stem

Go over the stem, and then underneath it, pulling back to the left. Pull upward, before going underneath the stem between the upper wraps and the lines that were laid by doing the securing of **steps 7 and 8**. From there, pull down, and finally push underneath the stem, pulling back to the left where we began.

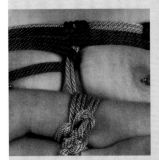

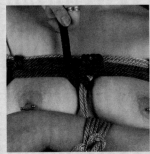

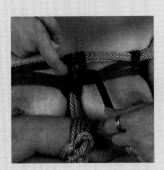

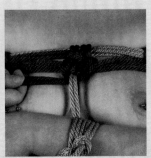

10

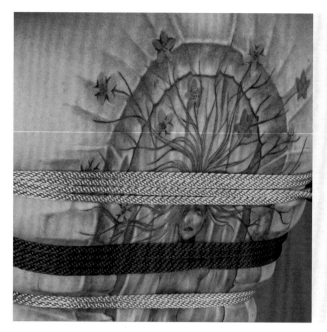

Wrap twice around the body

Wrap once around the body to the left, slightly below the last set of chest wraps. Place the second of these wraps directly beneath the one placed before it, without crossing the lines over one another. In this image, this set of wraps is shown in dark green.

Lock the stem - Part 1

Locking the stem follows a similar pattern as before. The rope comes from the right, goes over the stem, and comes under the stem returning to the right. Next, it is pulled up, before going underneath the stem in the space just below the place where we previously locked the stem. The rope is pulled down, before going one last time under the stem, heading back to the right.

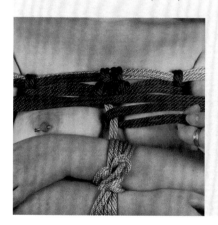
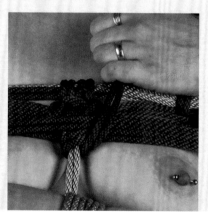
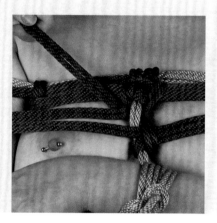

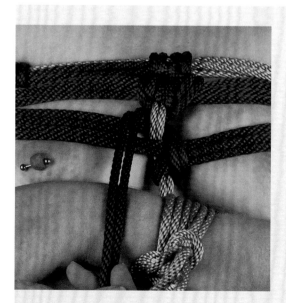
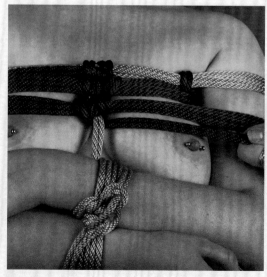

Lock the stem Part 2

The rope is pulled down, before going one last time under the stem, heading back to the right. Take the time once the stem is locked to push the lock upward, thus stabilizing the tie as well as making room for the final lock in **step 14.**

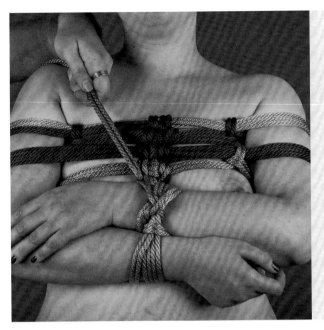

Secure wraps and lock the stem

Secure and hook right and left lower wraps. Repeat the technique shown in **steps 7-9**, securing and hooking the lower wraps.

Locking the stem follows a similar pattern as before. However, the knotwork might be getting a little snug in here. Manipulate the ropes by gently pushing the lines on the stem towards the top ropes.

The list of these details for locking off the stem a final time is the same as those described in **step 10**.

14

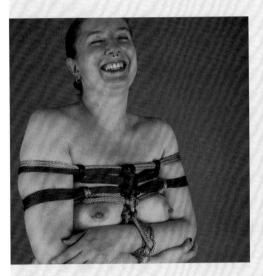

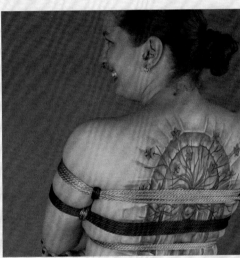

Tie off

Wrap around the stem enough times to create a solid line between the stem knots and the wrists, finally pulling through to create an overhand knot. The tension on the stem keeps the knots form slipping up and down, thus stabilizing the tie. Tighten down, and the tie is complete. Tuck in those loose ends, and you are good to go.

15

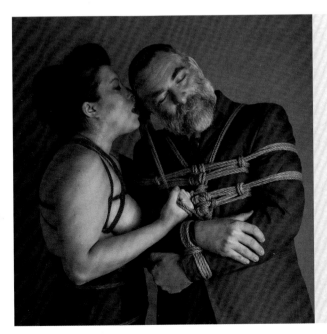

Once reconstructed entirely of jute rope, the finished result can look both like the tie shown at the beginning of the tutorial, or this variation with shoulder straps.

Exercise: One Piece of Rope

While learning different techniques for tying, it is important to get back to the basics—being with your partner and connecting through rope. At the end of the day, it isn't about the flashy detail ties or the contorted poses. It is about the two of you together, being present, being connected. It is about setting an intention together, having shared why you are into rope bondage, and what you get out of it. Rope, like the individual threads used to craft a tapestry, helps us weave something that is all ours.

Getting back to the basics also means seeing what you can do with a single piece of rope. So many Riggers get caught up with having heaping piles of rope and having all of the fancy techniques ready to go. Set it all aside for a moment. When you learn how to work with only one piece of rope, it will not matter what you tie. That piece of rope becomes a tool for transmission from your heart to theirs, and even a basic cuff will become a deeply connecting experience.

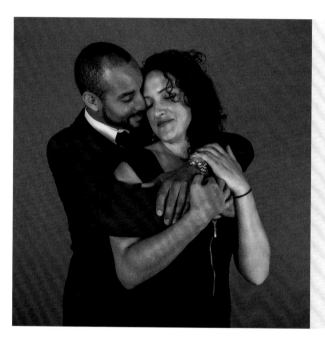

Connect

Before you pick up the rope, or perhaps with your rope curled up in one hand, hold your partner. Rest your head against them, or take a moment to have them sit at your feet with your hand on their shoulder. Let the dynamic of your relationship lead you, and be in the experience together.

1

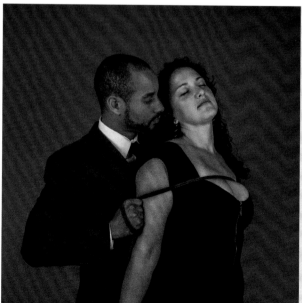

Pull a rope firmly around their body

This can be done with them facing you or with your body pushed up against their back. Pull them into you. Hold them tight using this piece of line as an extension of your will.

2

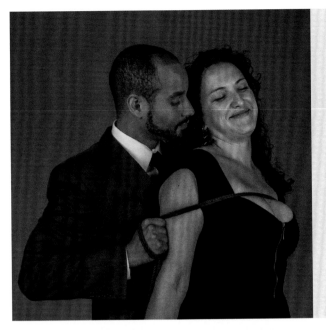

Inspire

This is a chance to energetically dance with your partner. Slowly slide the rope across their skin, letting it run across their chest, softly up to their neck, and come down once more. They might push back, pull in, or grab the rope themselves. Provide them with information about the emotion you want to inspire by pressing your body into them, winking, letting hands roam, or using seductive words. Some scenes are a waltz, and others a heated tango.

3

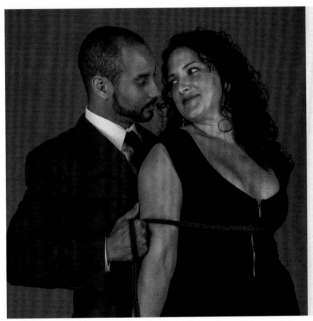

Look them in the eye

With the line still wrapped around them, catch their eye. Stop. With eyes locked, show your feelings towards them in that instant. The eyes are the windows to the soul, and in this moment connecting with rope, you can make a choice to open those windows wide.

4

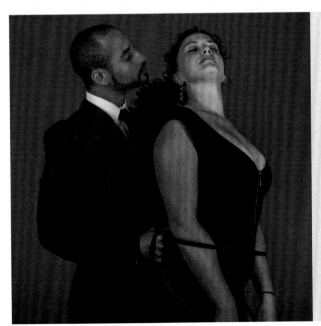

Express your passion

Whether that passion is erotic or joyous, feral or commanding, playful or sensual—show it. The rope will become a natural extension of that passion.

5

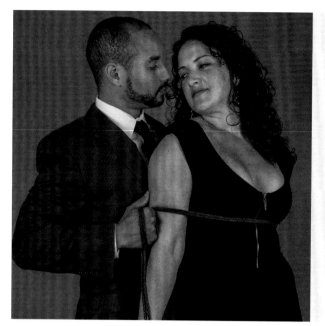

Be present

With the line still wrapped around them, catch their eye. Stop. With eyes locked, show your feelings towards them in that Remember as you follow this exercise that you are here, now, with them. You are not thinking about what you will do an hour from now, later in the scene, or what other projects need done in the rest of your life. You are here, now, with them, with this piece of rope. Both of you deserve the excellence of this moment, whatever it looks like.

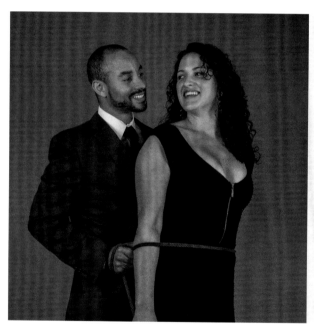

Be yourself

Be yourself in all your giggling and grandeur, in all of your seriousness and silliness. You can don characters for a scene if you like, because role-playing is fun. But at the end of the day, remember who you are. You don't have to tie rope or receive bondage like anyone else. Do it your way. Being authentic is sexy.

After the exercise, give each other some time to think about what you experienced. Some people need downtime to have space to let it all trickle through their systems. When you do share, remember that compassionate communication is key.

Own how you felt, what you experienced, rather than telling someone else what they experienced. Ask questions about what your partner experienced, rather than assuming you know what was going on in their head. Gift your partner with what will help the two of you have excellent scenes in the future, as compared to only getting frustrated about the past. It is important to lovingly be open about both, but make sure to share your joys, not just your challenges.

Whether we have thousands of feet of rope or a single line, intention and connection are tools that can last us a lifetime.

Facial and Detail Ties

Getting up close and personal can be hot and sexy, but it's also a great chance to interact with our partners in a more intimate way. With a tender hand, whether firm or delicate, we can spend literal face time with one another.

The face is one of the most intimate parts of our body to play with. We will often let strangers shake our hands, or even give us a hug, but our head is a precious thing indeed. Thus, binding of the face can feel very intense and profound, even if it is a simple gag or running a piece of rope along our partner's cheek.

For some of us, our faces come with stories of trauma. A slap across the face can be part of our history, or a fear embedded in us by our culture. Messing up makeup, being made to drool, or leaving indents on the face can trigger others. Something like a rope over the eyes can bring up feelings of helplessness. Kissing the eyelids or back of the ear lobes may be a kind of touch that your partner finds so intimate that they associate it with a special type of relationship.

Because of this, even more so than with bondage in general, it is important for a stream of communication to remain open when doing these sorts of ties. This can also mean debriefing after play, whether later that night, or days later. As there are some Bottoms who go nonverbal with some types of facial play because it can trigger an altered state of consciousness or "rope space," in-scene verbal communication may not be ideal. The post-scene conversation then becomes vital. Perhaps a partner's response was that of complete relaxation and comfort. What a great thing to know for the future!

Other parts of the body are also great for detail ties. The hair, hands, feet, genitals are all great chances for playing with areas of our Bottom's flesh that might not be used to receiving attention. Most often rope bondage focuses on larger segments of the body, and working on the small parts can put them in a different headspace. Explore, and see how these sorts of ties work into the play between you are your partner.

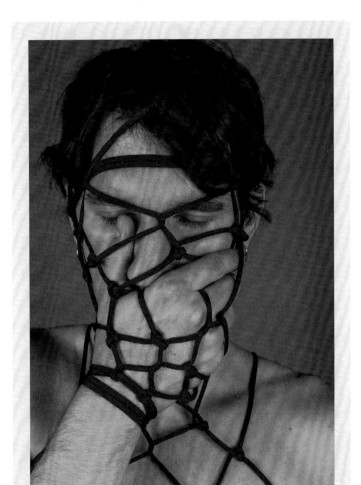

Facial bondage can be intricate, simple, or combined with other ties.

Bit Gag

This basic tie can be explored to muffle noise during a spanking, give our partner something to bite down on when they moan, or to engage in erotic embarrassment from the drool that may ensue. Consider tying this sheepshank knot in advance, like we did with the knot on the **Floral Harness.** By doing so you will be able to pull it out at a moment's notice.

But remember, once your partner is gagged, they will not be able to verbally communicate with you in the same way they were doing so before. Remember to discuss with your partner in advance about safety communication systems like hand squeezing, grunts, or dropping a bandanna, since they will not be able to use verbal safewords. Unless of course the two of you become fluent in each other's grunts and mumbles.

A 4-10ft (1-3 meter) piece of rope is perfect for a basic Bit Gag, using a material such as the nylon shown here.

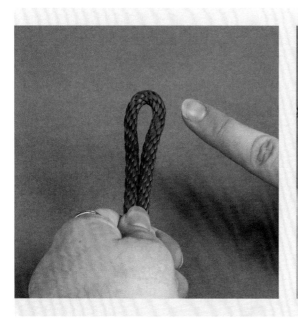
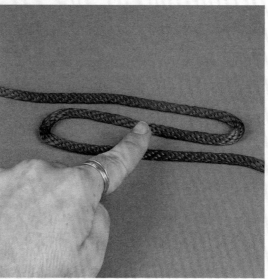

Create the letter "Z"

Place the center of your rope at the center of the middle line of the letter "Z." Each leg of the "Z" should be 3-4 inches (7-10 cm) long for most mouths. Doing this on a table is much easier, but you can try tying the bit gag (also known as a sheepshank knot) in the palm of your hand.

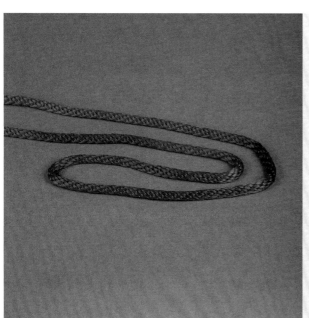

Loop the right side around

Bring the lower rope up and over the top of the right side. This will create two concentric curves on the right side.

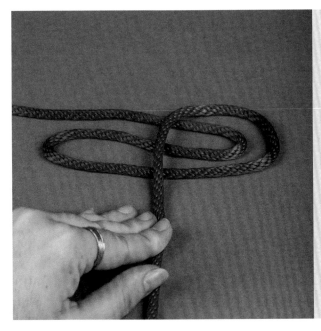

Lay over all lines

Create the letter "P" by using the running end of the right side rope and pointing it downward.

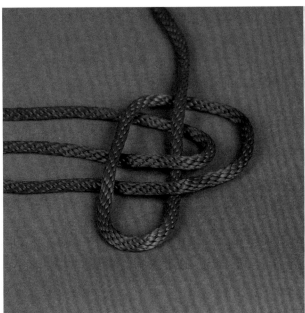

Tuck and bring up

Take the running end of the rope and tuck it under the bottom two lines, and bring forward in the gap between the top one and bottom two lines.

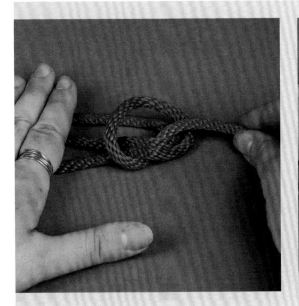 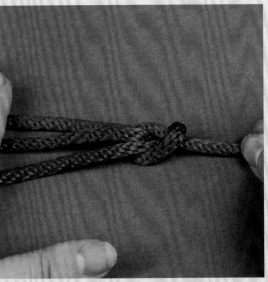

Tighten down

Hold the lines on the left side of the "Z," while pulling the running end on the right side with your right hand. The knot will collapse down into this shape.

Repeat

Repeat steps 2-5 on the left side, now with the wrap being under the left side of what was the "Z", and the tuck being brought up. You now have a completed sheepshank knot! Now we get to turn this into a bit gag.

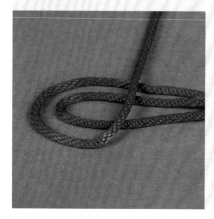 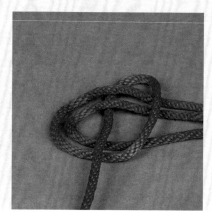 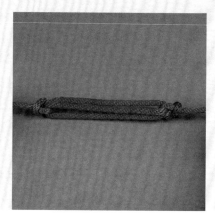

Insert gag

Place in the mouth, with two lines in the mouth, and one line below the chin to constrain the face further. You can also choose to insert all three lines in the mouth.

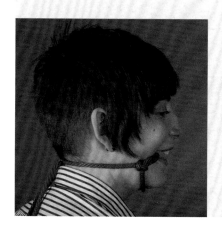 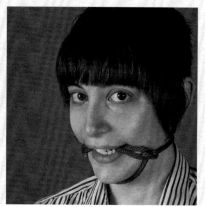 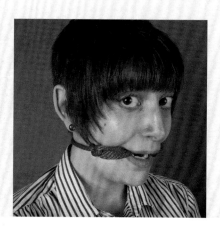

Insert gag

Tie in the back with a square knot, as snug as possible.

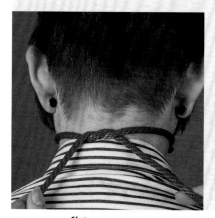 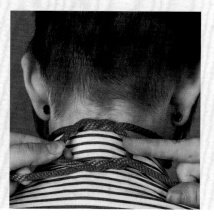 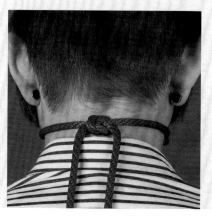

Hair Tie

Just as we mentioned in Chapter 2, there are a wide variety of columns available to tie and the hair can be one of them. It lets bondage enthusiasts also enjoy hair pulling. This tie is great for binding hair 4 inches (10 cm) or longer. For shorter hair, consider binding the head with a head cage and pulling on it. To pull hair specifically, Bottoms who enjoy intense sensations may enjoy the of use outside props like medical forceps and other sorts of clamps.

Silky or fine hair may hold rope better when it has product in it (such as hairspray, mousse, or gel), or by using a line that has more grip to it (such as jute). You can choose all of the hair on the head as a ponytail, half of the hair as a pigtail, or just a small amount. The smaller the amount of hair, the more challenging it may be for the person whose scalp it is, and the thinner width of line you may want to use.

This tie is being done with a 6ft (2 meter) piece of paracord.

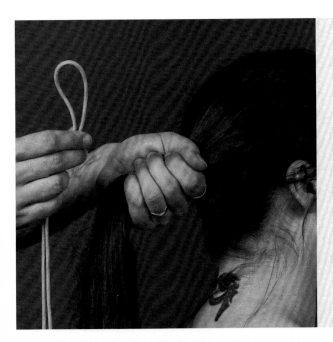

Gather hair and find the bight

Bring the hair you will be binding together into one hand, pulling with even tension in the directing you want it to be pulled in the final tie. Having done so, fold your rope in half.

1

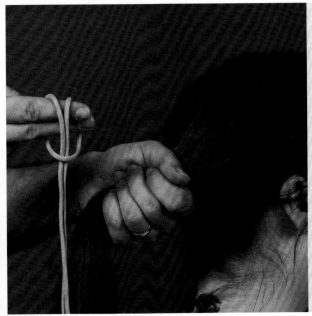

Create a lark's head

Take your folded rope and turn it into a lark's head knot, as shown in the tie used to add on additional rope featured earlier in this book for **adding rope** (see page 50).

2

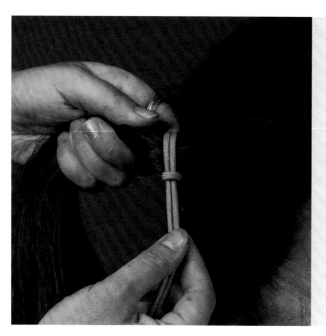

Slide lark's head onto hair

Take the bundle of hair and slide the lark's head as close to the hairline as possible. Wherever the lark's head is placed will be near where the final tie will sit.

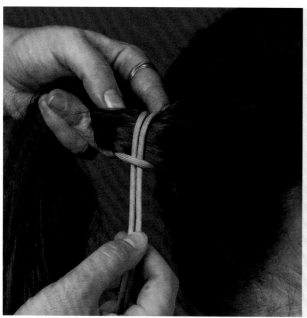

Open the lark's head up

Lay it flat along the hair.

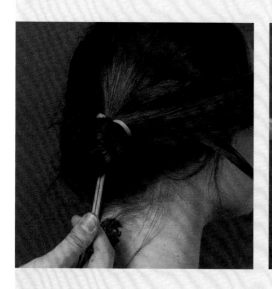
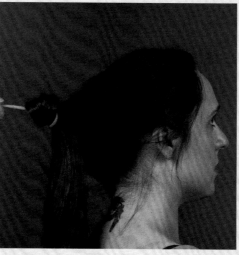

Fold the hair

Take the bundle of hair and fold it back on itself. The fold in the hair will be at the center of where the lark's head has been split open. Pull down with all of the folded hair in one hand, and the paracord in the other. The tie will slide to where the hair has been folded. Steps 2-5 shown in this Hair Tie are identical to those shown for **adding rope.**

Create loop

Grab onto the bundle of hair just below the fold (where the center of the paracord is located) with one hand. With the other hand, place three fingers underneath the loose line, pointing away from you. Bring your three fingers down and grab the line that was hanging down. Continue rotating the three fingers, with them next pointing at yourself (now holding the line), and then facing away from you once more. The line of paracord has now become a loop.

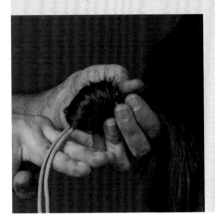
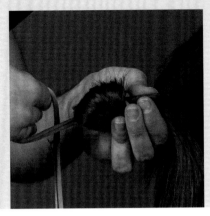
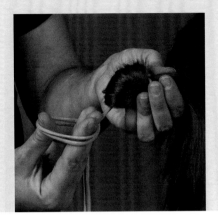

6

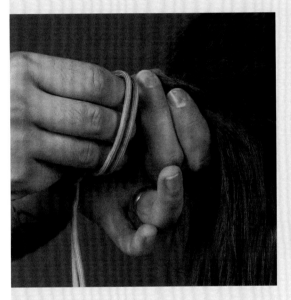
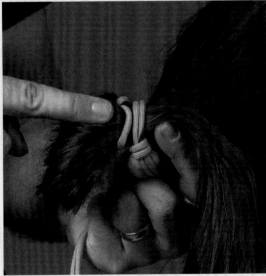

Slide loop

Slide the loop of paracord over the folded hair. Slide it just beyond the original point where the paracord was attached, closer towards the scalp. Tighten down firmly.

7

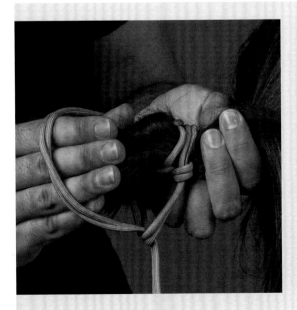
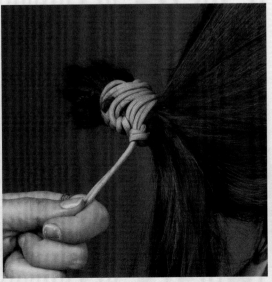

(optional) Place additional loops

Follow the pattern for **steps 6 and 7,** placing the loops closer and closer to the scalp. Though some hair and line combinations can work with a single loop over the lark's head, more loops are encouraged.

8

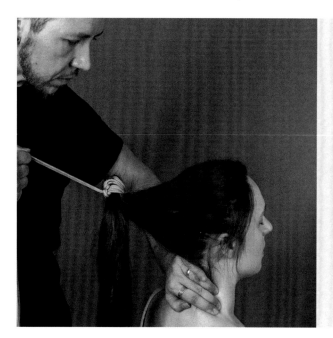

Slowly pull

Test out your bondage, while placing a hand on the back of their neck to avoid undue strain. You will note that the bondage slips down to the point in the hair where the hair was folded. Thus, if the folding was not tightly done, the bondage can slide away from the scalp, and perhaps even slide off completely.

Make sure to check in with your partner as you play with this tie. Attaching this tie to another body part might be sexy for a short period of time, but it could become be painful to their neck over time. An example of this might be tying hair down to their wrists behind the back, and then having the arms get tired. As their arms relax, more and more stress is placed on the neck.

Do not have a partner stand during this tie with the hair being the only line attached to the ceiling. If they were to pass out, their entire body weight would be held by only their hair, potentially causing serious body trauma. There are plenty of fun ways to play with hair bondage that do not endanger our partner.

Head Cage

Considered an advance technique by some, Head Cages can actually be broken down into a handful of simple steps. The same can be said for most forms of bondage. Next time you are looking at images of ropework, try deconstructing the images in your mind by seeing with ropes are on top. Those pieces of bondage were most likely tied last during the scene. Even the most complex ties are made out of simple steps.

When it comes to the head cage, the delicate nature of this tie requires all parties to slow down and become more aware of what they are doing. As a Bottom, close your eyes for much of the tie—not just to avoid a loose end hitting you somewhere painful, but to focus on where the lines are moving and feel the sensation fully. Letting the material dance over your skin can be a luscious treat. Tops are encouraged to go slowly and tenderly with this form of bondage, though using a delicate or firm hand is up to personal choice.

The tie shown is being executed with a 20ft (7 meter) piece of paracord.

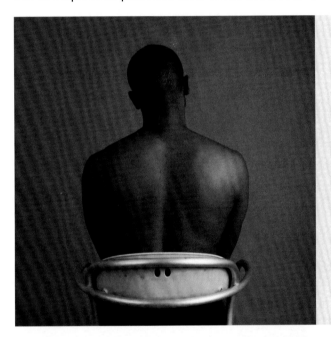

Have the bottom sit

Though this is an optional step, I find that trying to tie a Head Cage above the chest height of the Rigger can be taxing on the Rigger's body. Having a Bottom sit allows both partners to be more comfortable during the tie, which is especially important in complex Head Cages that may take a while to complete. Binding a partner to a chair, having them kneel, or be bound in some other way can help the time involved in this tie be part of a scene.

1

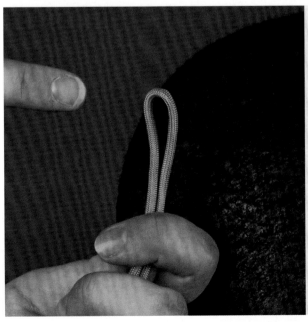

Find the bight

Fold your rope in half.

2

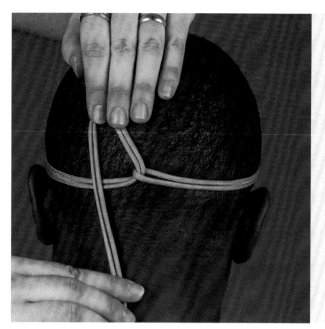

Create lark's head

Wrapping around the head half an inch (1-2 cm) above the eyebrows, pull the long end of the rope through the bight. Having done so, pull the rope in a direction that creates reverse tension (gets tighter) above the head-wrap line, and let the loose end fall.

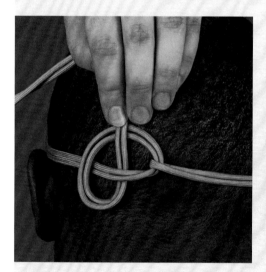

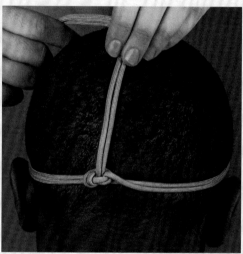

Tie half hitch knot

To secure the forehead wrap by reaching your fingers (the ones that are not holding open the triangle from step 4 open) under the forehead wraps down through the triangle shown. Pull the line upwards, and then hold the forehead wrap at the lark's head bight as you tighten down the half hitch knot. The forehead line should be able to have two fingers slide underneath it, but not be falling off.

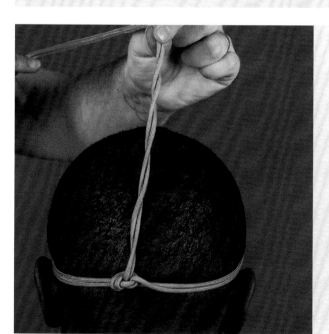

Twist

Take the line and twist it four to eight times. This will be the piece that later is split apart to add security on the top of the head, and be available to tie into for more complex head harnesses. Run the twisted lines across the center of the head.

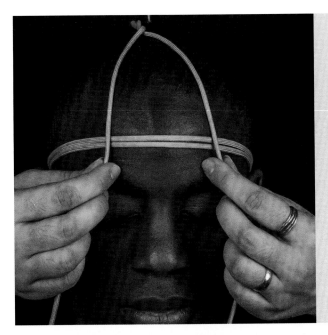

Split the line

Once you get to the hairline, split the pair of lines apart. This example is shown with me standing behind the Model, but it is often easier to do the tie when Rigger and Model are face to face.

6

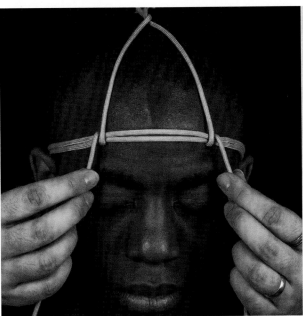

Wrap the forehead lines

Lay the left line over the forehead lines, then pull it up under on the outside of the split line. Lay the right line on the opposite side, pulling it up under on the outside of the split line.

7

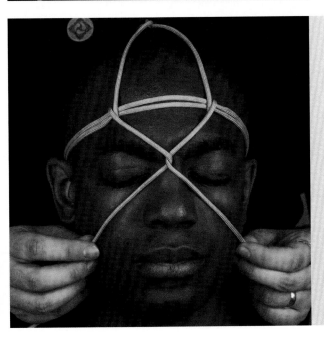

Twist at the nose

At the bridge of the nose, twist the ropes around each other, continuing down along the angle of the cheek.

8

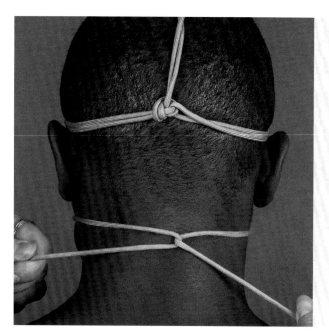

Twist at the back

At the back of the head, twist at the nape of the neck.

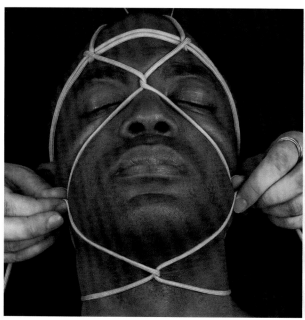

Twist under the chin

Bringing the line forward once more, twist under the chin. Make sure the twist is above the Adam's apple, and is loose enough not to impact blood flow or breathing.

Lock at left cheek line

Bring the left rope up, lay the rope across the cheek line, and then pull it back down on the outside, closer to the ear. Cross the line just laid, and then bring the rope up under the cheek line on the side closer to the nose. Locking off in this manner is also referred to as tying a Munter hitch.

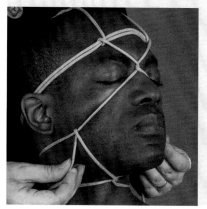 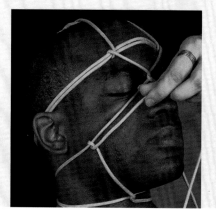 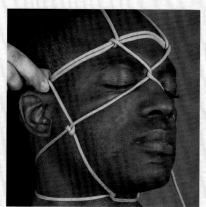

Lock the forehead lines

Bringing the left rope up, lay the rope over the forehead line half an inch (1-2 cm) from the ear, pulling it back down on the outside of where you came up. Cross the line just laid, and then bring the rope up under the forehead line on the side further from the ear. In doing so you have created another Munter hitch. Repeat on the right side of the face.

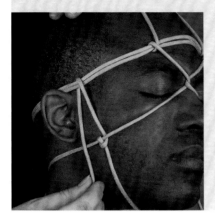
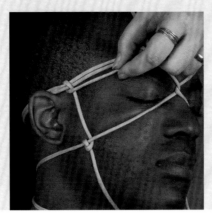
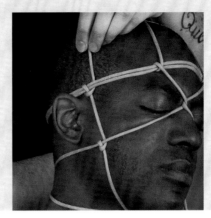

Catch the center line

Split the center line on the top of the head apart between twists. Pull the ropes underneath (from bottom to top) the area that has been split open, snugging the head harness down. Pull the ropes towards the forehead before doubling back, this time underneath the lines that were just laid.

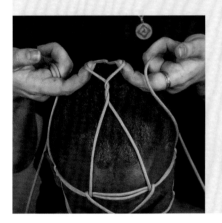
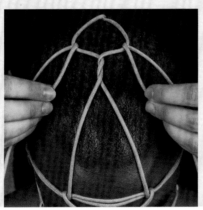
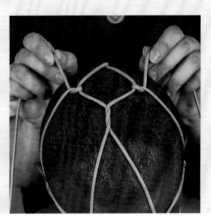

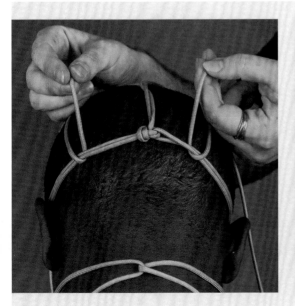
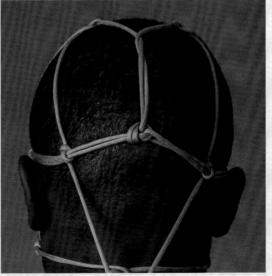

Lock the forehead line

As you come across the line at the back of the head, create a Munter hitch on each side.

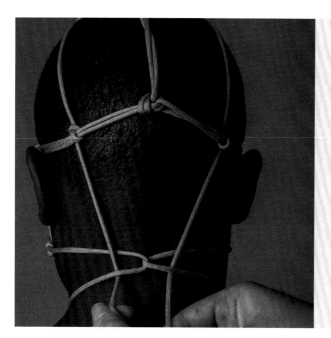

Pull underneath lowest lines

Take the lines down and tuck underneath the lowest chin/neck wraps.

15

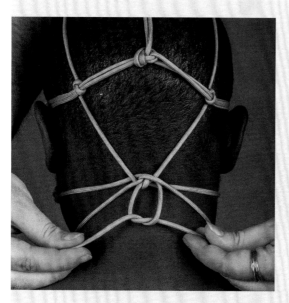

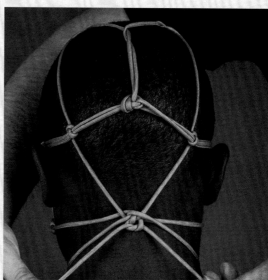

Lock the forehead line

As you come across the line at the back of the head, create a Munter hitch on each side.

16

The finished tie, having taken the loose ends and twisted them around, looks like this:

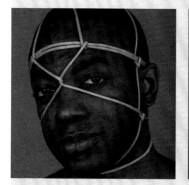

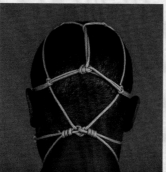

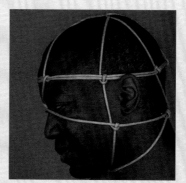

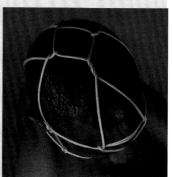

Once you have practiced the version shown here, explore being creative, and have fun! Some examples are shown below, but the sky is the limit. You can also play around with other materials, such as yarn, cross-stitch thread and lace. Leather cording can be a fun option for the leather fetishists among us, or thin jute line for those who love the smell of it. Remember though, this can leave marks on the face. Make sure not to play right before heading to a family gathering or an office party.

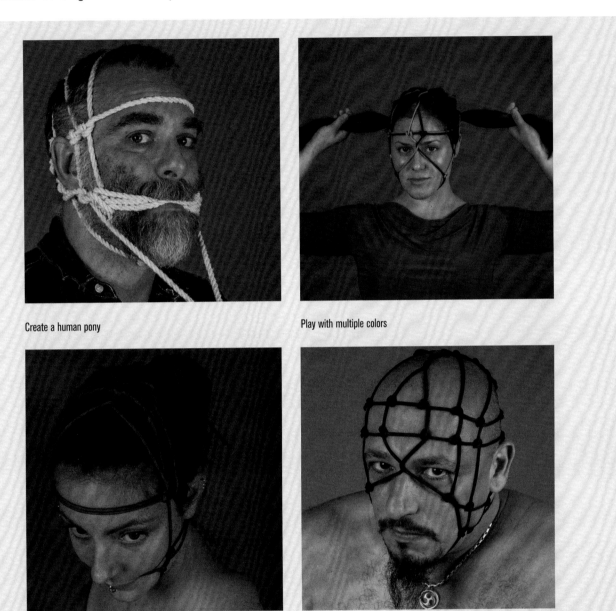

Create a human pony

Play with multiple colors

Incorporate hair bondage

Enjoy being fierce

Hand Harness

This same sort of twisting and weaving can be used on other parts of the body to create intricate harnesses and cages. In this variation, the hand is chosen for framing. But at home, try playing around with these techniques on the feet, external genitalia, boots, or whatever else tickles your fancy.

In the case of a foot, bind the base framework around the ankle. For external genitals, gently lift up the cock and balls, tying around both. In both cases, be careful. Tightening down hard around the feet can become painful and can lead to cramping or breaking of tiny bones in the foot if the Bottom stands. Avoid twisting the balls around each other when tying, which can be excruciating and damaging.

Some people are incredibly ticklish! I've seen Bottoms accidentally lash out and hit their Tops because of a rope running between their toes. And as for genital ties, pulling out pubic hairs is unlikely to earn you friends.

A 10ft (3 meter) piece of paracord is being used to craft this tie.

Create base for framework

Follow **steps 2-5** from the **Head Cage** (see page 69) to wrap the doubled line around the wrist, create a lark's head, and tie off with a half hitch knot. Leave one or two finger's worth of slack underneath the wrist bindings, as the harness will snug up with each step in the tie.

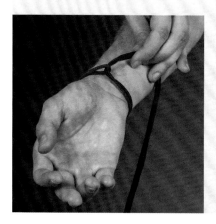 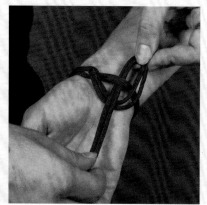 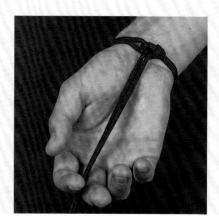

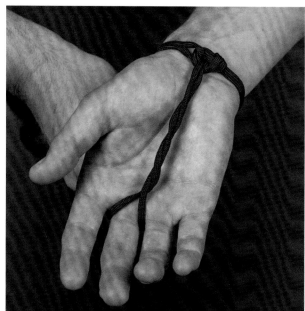

Twist and split

Take the line and twist it three to six times. Run the twisted lines down the center of the palm, and split the line apart to run with one strand on each side of the middle finger.

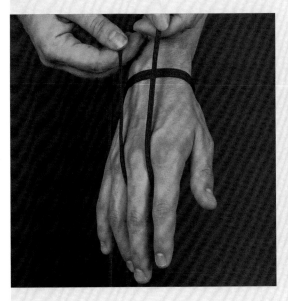
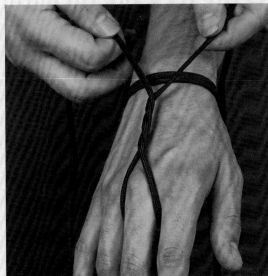

Twist again

Take the line and twist it three to six times, running the line down the back of the hand.

3

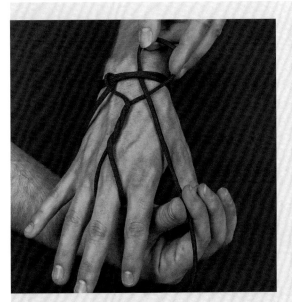
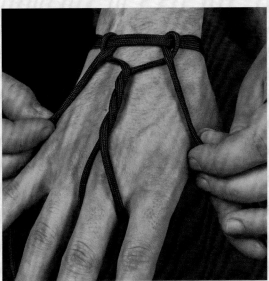

Wrap the wrist cuff

Crossing over the wrist cuff, take the right strand and pass it back under the wrist cuff on the side closer to the center of the wrist. Repeat on the left side as a mirror image of the right side. Slide the lines an inch (2.5 cm) apart.

4

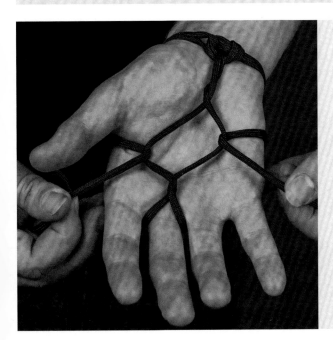

Catch the palm line

Split the palm line between twists. Pull the ropes underneath (from bottom to top) the area that has been split open, slightly snugging the hand harness down.

5

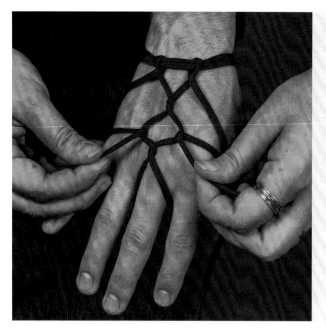

Catch the back of hand line

Split the lines at the back of the hand between twists. Pull the ropes underneath (from bottom to top) the area that has been split open, slightly snugging the hand harness down.

Tie off

On the left side, tie an overhand knot around the nearest line to the free strand of paracord while keeping the harness snug. Repeat on the right. This will leave a symmetrical diamond pattern on the back of the hand, just as was done on the palm of the hand.

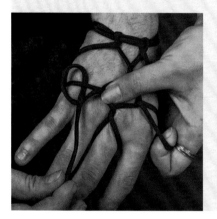 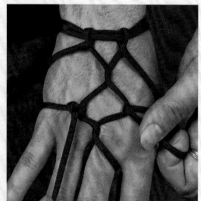 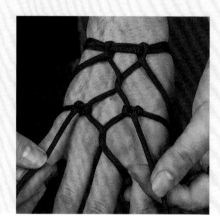

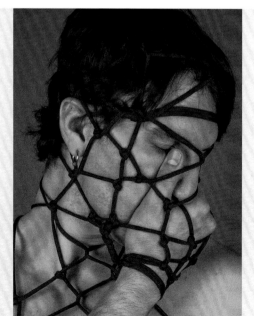

(optional) Attach

At this point the Hand Harness is finished. However, with the two loose ends on the back of the hand, there are many choices for attaching the hand to another piece of bondage. It can be tethered to a chest harness to force someone to hold their own breasts. The tie can be bound to a crotch rope for sexual delight. In this case, the Hand Harness was attached to the **Head Cage** (see page 69) to create a gag made of the Model's own body part.

Cutting Your Rope

With facial bondage, there are individuals who may get claustrophobic or have other emotional responses, which may require quickly releasing our partners from bondage. Removing ropes efficiently with calm confidence is very important. Much of the time, a situation that looks like a rope might need to be cut can be taken care of by untying the ropes with that same calm confidence. Holding a partner still, looking them in the eyes, and breathing slowly while telling them that you are going to remove the ropes now, can reduce the stress for the bound partner. This gives the Rigger plenty of time to remove the restraints from the Model's body.

Take a deep breath, and methodically untie. Work the steps backwards from what got the tie into place. If Tops begin to lose their cool, it only exacerbates any situation at hand. Untying rope in situations of duress can actually help bring partners together and show that the trust a Bottom was giving was well founded when it is done with grace and composure. This is important to remember because there is a belief by some Bottoms that if they use a safeword, the bondage will be instantly done. This is not the case. It will take time to untie.

However, having the option for cutting rope is important. Cutting the rope off, without blame on anyone's part, can allow us to move forward to tie another day... or even later that night. Getting back on the horse, for

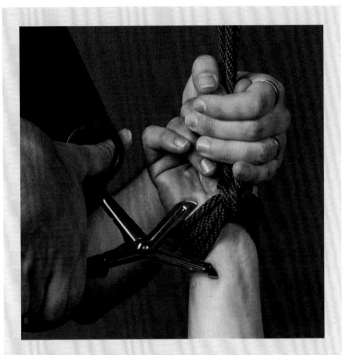

NEVER point a blade at your partner's skin when cutting ropes.

some people (on either side of the rigging) can curb the unfounded fears and internal stories of inadequacy that might otherwise arise from having to cut rope or quickly untie a partner. You can replace your rope, but your partner is irreplaceable.

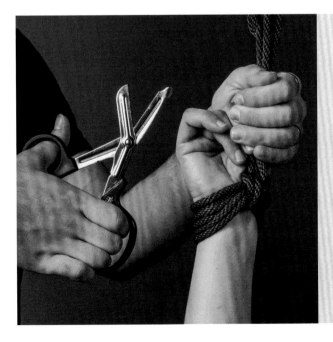

Grab your shears

Have your shears or cutting tool nearby. There are a wide variety of tools to choose from, and which you choose to have is up to you.

1

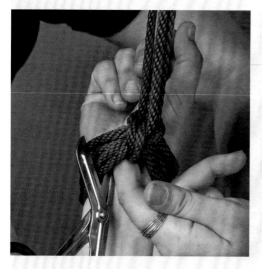 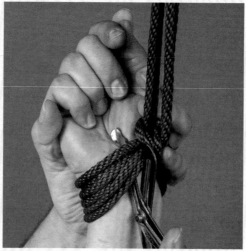

Pull ropes out

Pull the ropes away from the body. Carefully slide the cutting tool underneath the rope, making sure to angle it away from the skin. Cut the line while making sure your partner will not squirm and hurt themselves, for example using your other hand to immobilize the limb. This is especially important on the face, or near sensitive areas of the body.

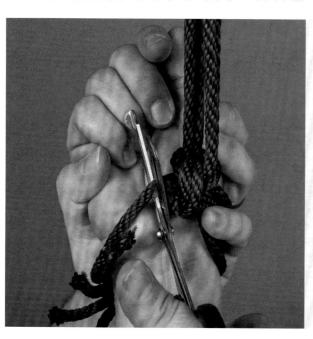

Cut all lines

Make sure to cut through all of the lines associated with the tie. Not doing so may cause the bondage to tighten down onto the remaining strands, increasing pain and potentially causing damage.

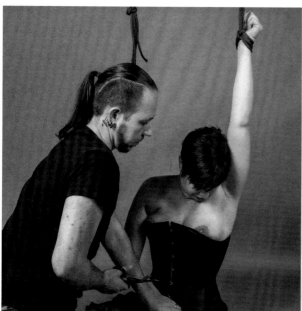

Release limbs

Having removed the ropes while staying cool, release the unbound limb. If the Model is panicking, consider holding the limb that has been released so they do not harm themselves.

Cut off ropes and support body

Cut all ropes necessary. If the challenge is with their wrists, you do not need to cut off the crotch rope—only cut off the ropes related to the issue. Use the frame of your body to support the weight of anyone who is unconscious, making sure to keep their head from hitting the ground.

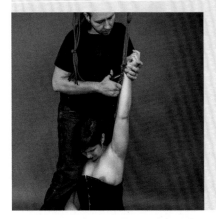
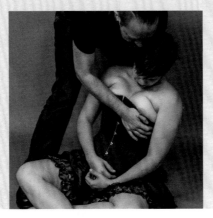
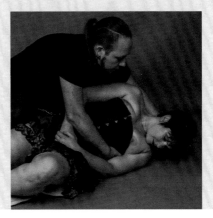

5

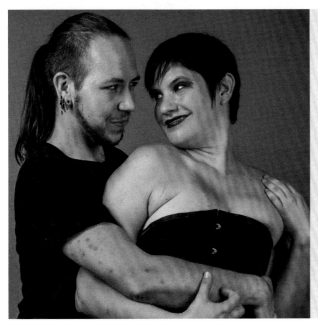

Reconnect

Make sure to take the time with your partner to reconnect after ropes have been cut, or if anything did not go as originally planned. Whether you play again, cuddle, have sex, or spend time in casual conversation is up to you. This is not a time for intense processing, let alone blame. If in doubt, consider grabbing a glass of water, warming up their body, and asking what else each of you needs.

6

Seek medical assistance where there is any concern about joint injury, circulation, nerve damage, etc. Hospitals have seen a variety of injuries before, and the shoulder strain from a hand pulled upward and back with a rope does not have different care needs than an injury from a variety of sports activities. If the issue of your kinky play arises, make sure that both partners are clear with their health care providers about the consensual nature of your fun. Their concern may be amplified if your stories do not match, or it seems like a lie is taking place. This is especially true if there are marks, bruises and abrasions on the flesh.

Though these concerns are unlikely in rope play, it is wise to plan for the best and prepare for the worse. Being aware of what medical issues might arise and knowing what to do in such emergencies helps our partners know we care.

Exercise: Running Hands Over Rope

Taking the time to experience the sensation of the rope while it is on the skin is an opportunity to create more depth in bondage scenes. Exploring the range of tactile information available to us, we explore each other's bodies and reactions as well. This is especially important to remember with facial bondage, but applies to all forms of rope play that we do.

It is important to remember that the exercises we are trying in this book can build a high degree of intimacy between play partners. I mention this because there are Tops and Bottoms alike who are used to their bondage, kink and sex lives being mechanical, or only involving sexual intimacy. Putting a partner's every reaction at the forefront of our awareness may be the first time someone ever really "saw" us. This can be experienced as "love" by some play partners and lead to what is called "new relationship energy." Make sure to communicate with a play partner before and after a scene as to whether this sort of emotional connection is desired or not.

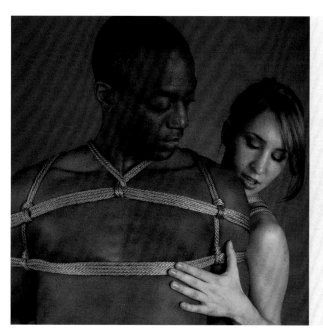

Apply rope

Take time to put rope on your partner. This can be restrictive or decorative rope, out of any material that strikes your fancy. Feel free to put rope on yourself as well if it makes you or your partner happy.

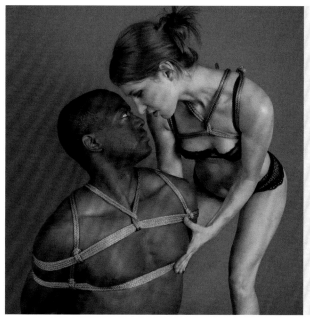

Almost touch

Enjoy the art of the tease. Whether it is a kiss, a stroke, a thud, or a bite... almost do it. Do so by getting within an inch (2.5 cm) of their skin and then pull back. This can help charge both of you up for the rest of the exercise, building up heat and desire.

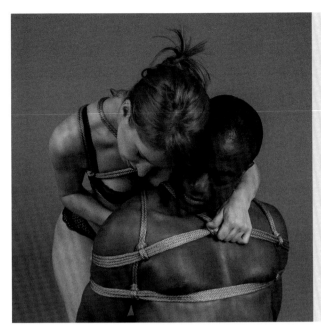

Grab the ropes

Slide your hands under the ropes and pull on them. If they are precariously balanced, make sure to support their body. Let them know you have control of them. The firmness pushes the rope into them—creating tension, creating a new sensation.

3

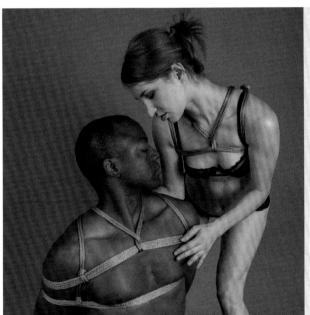

Touch only their skin

Find the empty spaces between ropes. Run fingers or palms over those spaces, avoiding the rope. Remind them (verbally or non-verbally) that they have granted you permission to access their flesh, and that they are exposed in this moment. If their body is covered in clothing, run your hands along their forehead, neck and fingertips.

4

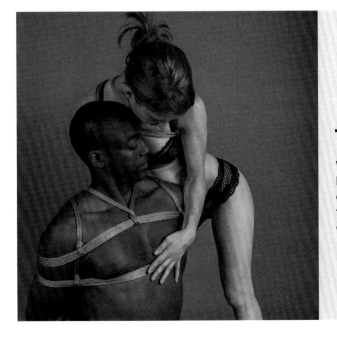

Touch only the ropes

With delicate fingers or a firm hand, touch only the lines you have laid. Avoid their skin. Try different levels of pressure and see how each of you respond when compared to the experience before of touching only their skin. Exploring the ropes with your lips can also cause interesting reactions for some Tops and Bottoms.

5

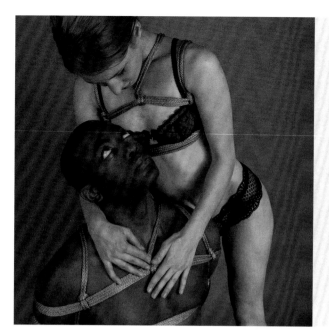

Touch both at the same time

Take the palm of your hand and run it over both the rope and their skin at once. Compare the sensations. Do this over the rest of their body, seeing how they respond. Offer them the full quality of your touch, not just quantity. Experiment with doing this step with the Rigger looking at the ropes, and with the Rigger looking in the eyes of the Model.

At this point, you can return to the rest of your scene, or continue with exploring both the rope and their flesh. Let your hands trace lines down to other parts of their body before adding rope to that region. Take off the ropes and caress the indents left behind. Licking the ropes, exposed skin, skin about to be bound, or indents left behind can also be a sexy way for some bondage explorers to enjoy one another.

Though shown using ties that cover larger areas on the body, this exercise is delectable for detail ties. Try running a fingertip between the thinnest of lines on a head cage, or between the webs formed in hand ties. Seeing the reactions to the same techniques on the torso or legs compared to touching the ears and thumb can be fascinating. Adding a blindfold to this exercise can also enhance the sensations for some Bottoms.

Rope and Erotic Power

Erotic restraint is full of opportunities to express power dynamics and dominant/submissive roles. Whether or not you are interested in dominance and submission, this chapter can help you find ideas you can use to "pervert" your rope play.

Rope has power. Rope is a living thing. It can be woven into body harnesses and corsets for decoration of the form. It can be braided into a whip to exact discipline onto waiting flesh. Rope can become a leash, a blindfold, a gag, a circle for creating sacred space.

Because of the versatility of rope, it has the capacity to be used for so many different sets of intentions, as examined in Chapter 1. But many people look at rope bondage and ask "when can we get to the good stuff," implying that rope is only a means to an end. But sometimes, rope is the point. Rope can be done for the sake of rope.

As a tool for the consensual exchange of erotic power, rope takes on a special meaning. A pair of handcuffs can be slapped on haphazardly, but rope bondage gives us the opportunity to be conscious whenever we play. We are showing an act of intention and consciousness, because we craft our bondage anew each and every time. The chances for diving into erotic dominance and submission (also known as D/S) start to ripple to the surface as lines dig into flesh and the sensual caress of a piece of jute across the skin takes hold.

Rope as ritual, rope as a way to build trust, rope as an expression of will. Rope as power exchange is not about specific ties, but about the focus brought to the bondage and the way it is carried out.

Even if you do not think that erotic power exchange is a part of your path in bondage, the following chapter will give ideas as to how to move your partner, untie your rope as part of your scene, and more. Who knows, something might jump out at you that you were not previously aware of having an interest in.

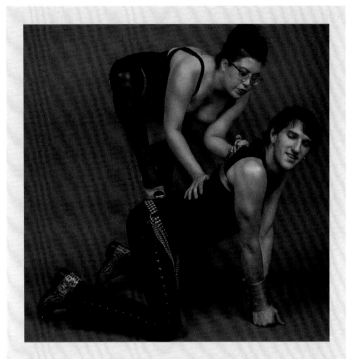

Find your own form of dominance, and your own style of submission.

Prep for Success

For energetic exchange to flow, it is useful to prepare the path ahead. If we are pulling a heavy cart down a road, it is easier to make sure the road is clear in advance, rather than have to stop every 10 feet and move fallen branches or stones that we come across. Just as with pulling a cart, wc will never be aware of everything that will cross our road. But preparing in advance for what we can know about might help the connection between us be shared more smoothly. It can also let our partner know that we cared enough to take the time in advance to build an experience that all parties would enjoy.

Have your tools ready

Make sure your rope is in the room you want to play in. Check that your safety shears are somewhere easy to access. Grab a bottle of water (plus a straw to help a bound partner drink from it), and a protein bar or snack in case their body (or yours) has such needs. Know where your inhaler and allergy meds are.

But that is not all! Are the bamboo poles or specific furniture you might want to tie them placed where you want them? Are the blindfolds, gags, chopsticks, clips, whips, and other kinky toys in easy range? What about the condoms, dental dams, latex gloves, and lube you might want? Having it all arranged in advance can create a peace of mind for all parties involved, and means all parties can focus on each other rather than figuring out where your favorite vibrator might be.

Know your ties

Practice your ties in advance. Get to know them. Have practice sessions before you play, especially if your play will involve any form of solemnity. In many areas, there are groups that meet up and practice (see page 126), or you can practice at home. But you know what? Not everyone's play is solemn. Some joke and laugh... and that can be done from a place of submission and surrender as well. Each set of individuals is unique.

For those that enjoy tying complex knots as the starting place of your ties, consider practicing the tie by yourself

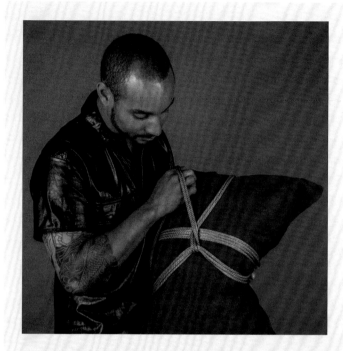

Wearing fetish gear while tying up your pillow is optional.

while listening to music or watching television. You might even come up with new knots when fooling around with your rope. If you are new to rope, a blindfold can go a long way towards setting the mood. They don't have to know that you are tripping over your own knots. You can pull on the ropes and pretend you "meant to do that."

Check in with their body, and yours

Have you eaten recently? What about hydration, or using the bathroom? These may sound like little things, but holding someone's trust in your hands while your stomach is gurgling is less than sexy. Check in with how both of you are doing emotionally as well. Events in the outside world might have us not want to play that night, or perhaps that stressful thing at work makes surrendering in bondage all the more appealing. This might be the perfect time for a moment of catharsis in your caring hands.

Keep Your Cool

Ever have those days where things just don't go as planned? The roommate comes home early? Ropes get all tangled up? Your back spasms? The cat starts chewing up your sex toys?

Keep your cool. Even in the worst situations, panicking or losing your temper does not help. Especially in the worst situations. By maintaining composure in the face of challenges that arise, you are able to support the framework of dominance in your rope scenes, and in general show you can be trusted with your Bottom's safety.

If your partner needs to be moved from a position, it does not benefit your power exchange or relationship as a whole to place blame. Bodies sometimes need to be moved. To say it is your partner's fault that the scene did not go as originally planned is a brutal way to destroy their ego and identity, as well as create alienation and emotional distress. The same can be said of stating that your dominant partner should have known to tie the bondage better. In the midst of a scene, most of us enter into an altered state of consciousness. Being told cruel things during this time can hit people much harder than it might otherwise.

If you need to break role during your power exchange encounter, it does not mean the Rigger cannot continue to guide the experience. Role-playing dominance can be a lot of sexy fun, but being in your authentic dominance introduces your partner to a part of your humanity they might not get to see otherwise.

Sometimes though, things go wrong. Injuries take place and feelings get hurt. Though keeping your cool may be appropriate, that does not mean avoiding responsibility. Apologizing and making amends is part of part of what makes someone an adult in healthy relationships. Engaging in power exchange dynamics, dominance, submission, or rope play does not negate that.

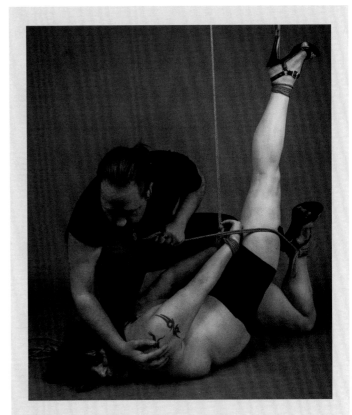

Even if the Top is panicking on the inside, keep breathing and stay calm.

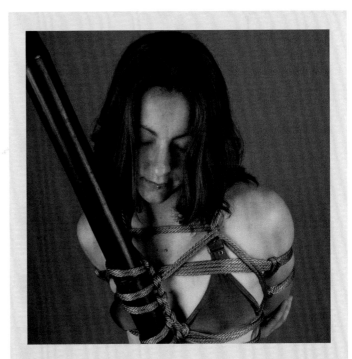

Binding someone as a work of art, or in an unusual position, can change their headspace.

Triskelion Crotch Rope

Just as power exchange is deeply personal, so is every person's relationship to their physical form. Some feel comfortable in it, and even enjoy flaunting it nude for the masses. Others have problems with having their partners touch them, especially in intimate places.

For these reasons, crotch ropes can be a tool of intimacy for many, and power exchange for others. In D/S, this can be an act of claiming, letting their partner know this region is theirs to possess, use, and delight in. They enjoy this gift of possession that has been given freely and consensually. Showing respect for a partner's discomfort can display power through compassion.

This decorative lower body tie starts with a matching knot to the **Floral Harness** (see page 44). Instead of a five-sided knot, it makes a three-sided knot in a similar style, thus deriving the name "Triskelion" from the interlocking swirls found in the classical motif.

This tie is done with 10-20ft (3-7 meter) of rope, depending on the frame of the individual being bound.

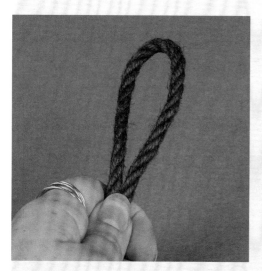
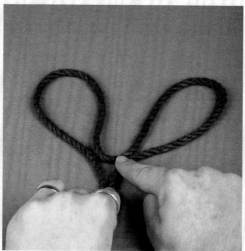

Create two petals

Lay the lines out on the ground or table. Each of the "petals" of this Triskelion knot can be between 6-18 inches (15-46 cm). The middle of the rope is pictured here as the lowest point between the petals.

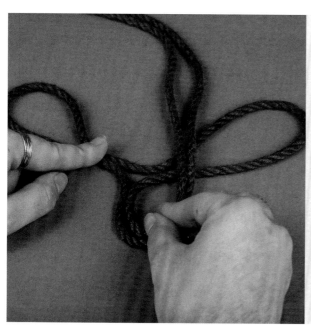

Lay lines counterclockwise

Beginning with the long ends, lay the lines over the next set of ropes or petal.

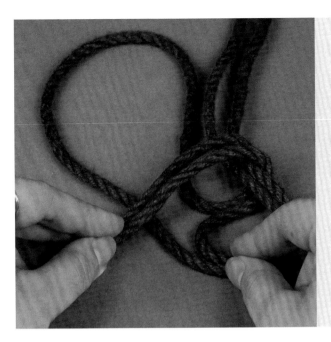

Repeat

Repeat step 2 with the next set of lines, crossing over the line that was just laid and the next petal.

3

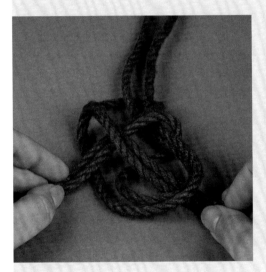 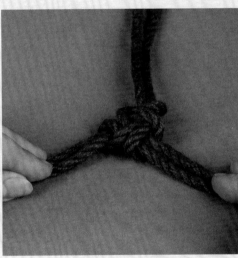

Lay and tuck under

Repeat the clockwise laying over with the third petal, crossing over the line that was just laid, then tucking underneath the first petal (the one with the loose ends). This will create a complete circle of ropes. Slowly tighten down each petal a bit at a time. If you find there are twists in your lines as you tighten, take the time to untwist them to make sure the knot lays flat.

4

Reverse directions

Beginning with the loose ends, lay over each set of ropes, this time clockwise. On the third petal, tuck under the first petal to create the complete circle. Tighten down on the finished knot, applying even tension to each line as you go around, snugging each a bit at a time.

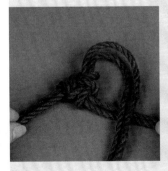 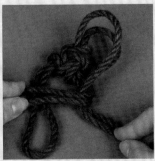 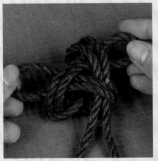 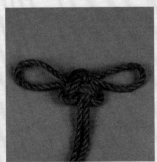

5

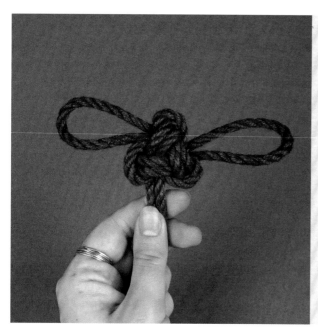

Flip over

You have now completed the **Triskelion knot**! Now let's get this onto our partner, shall we? And remember, feel free to tie this knot in advance and keep it stored in your rope bag to be able to skip straight to the next step during a scene.

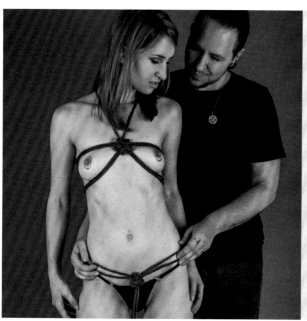

Center the knot

Place the knot on or just above the pubic mound. The loose ends will fall down between the legs. You can have your partner hold the knot in place, which creates a great opportunity for collaborative creativity, or hold it in place yourself.

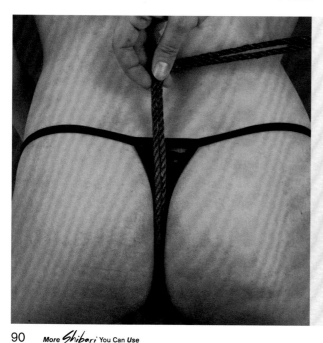

Between the legs

Run the loose ends up between the legs. Consider splitting the lines apart for individuals with external genitals, bringing the lines back together on the back side of the body.

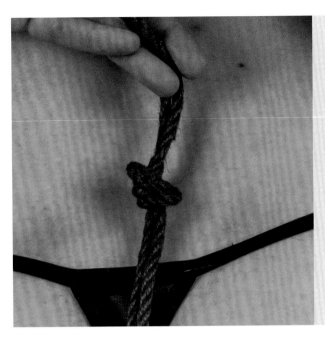

Overhand knot

Tie an overhand knot just below the waistline.

9

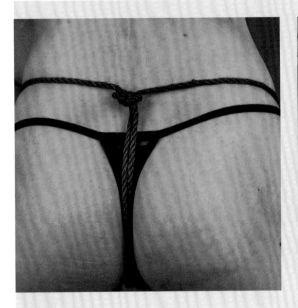

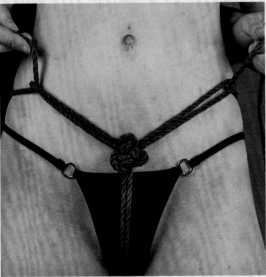

Run to the front and catch

Bring one of the loose ends onto each side of the hips, and "catch" the petals by running through them from bottom to top. The rope should lay on or just above the hips.

10

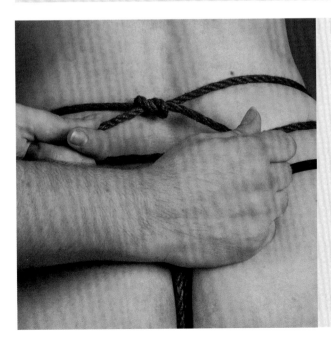

Bring to the back and tie off

Create the snugness you want in the finished tie as you pull the ropes back. Bring your ropes together and tie off with a square knot, reef knot, or other similar tie. Take a moment to hold your hand over the knot, or pull on it, to remind your partner of the connection between you.

11

Together the **Floral Harness** and **Triskelion Crotch Rope** make a delicate matched pair:

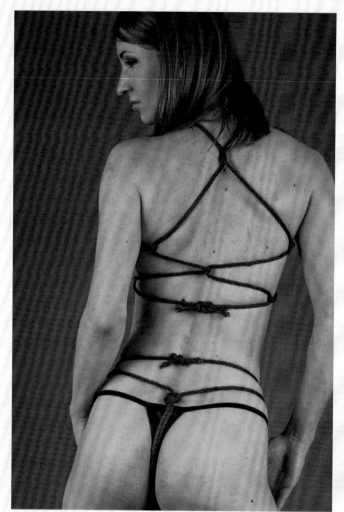 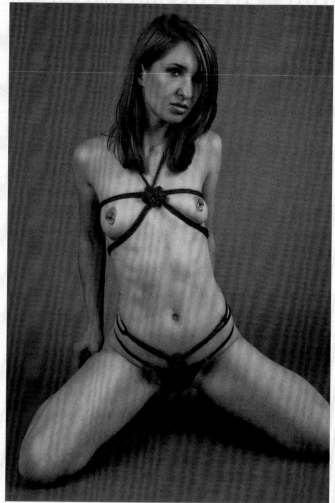

Keep Your Comfort

For some riggers, being physically at ease helps them be more watchful of subtle cues from their partner. Though this is not the case for everyone, body comfort can help many dominant partners focus on their Submissive.

Consider what you are wearing in a scene. Corsets, heels, tight leather clothing, and uniforms may be a fantastic option for fetishists, but they may or may not be needed for scenes between rope enthusiasts. Assumptions get made that unless the trappings of D/S and fetish pornography are in an encounter, the encounter is not "real." Ask your partner what turns them on. If the answer for both of you is that being nude, or in 1950's garb, or head-to-toe latex, or jeans and a flannel shirt is what is going to do it for you—do it. If you do choose to be nude it might even prove an advantage—bare feet means not accidentally standing on your own ropes!

Be aware of the comfort of your own body beyond the clothing. If you have problems with standing for too long, assume dominance by sitting in your throne and having your partner kneel before you. If you would prefer not to bind on the floor, what about investing in a massage table to tie them up on? Afterwards, as an act of service, they might be able to thank you with a massage.

To continue enforcing power dynamics after a scene, consider what aftercare would reflect that. Having a submissive partner curl up around our boots, bundle our ropes, or having them get water for both of you may give them a chance to come out of their altered state of awareness while still submitting to your will. This kind of connection can continue building emotional comfort in some relationships and play. For more about aftercare, see Chapter 7.

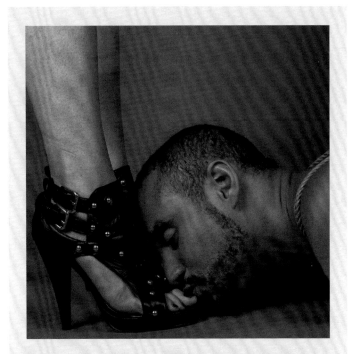

It might be sexy to wear heels when you tie, but will foot pain distract you?

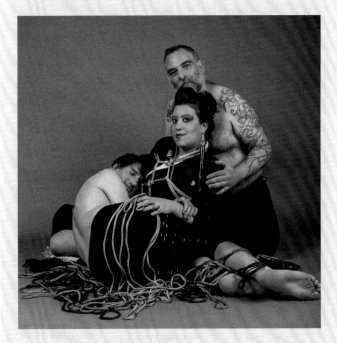

Even during aftercare, you can still maintain roles if desired.

Dominance and Submission

We all engage in power disparity in our lives, sometimes consciously, oftentimes unconsciously. We have power exchanges with our bank teller, our boss, and our family members.

One of the key differences that comes into kinky power play is consent. When we choose to be bound, we not only choose the ropes we use, but the person we play with, and how we will interact with them. Because we are doing this by choice (even when we choose to role-play struggling or "consensual non-consent"), we acknowledge the power that we have, and hand it over to our Rigger. We acknowledge the power we are receiving from our Model, and give it the respect it deserves. Instead of having power drained from only one side, the energy flows back and forth, charging the battery of both partners.

This consensual exchange requires trust on both sides—that our Top will take care of what we have handed over, and that our Bottom will share everything we need to know about what has been handed over. When the person being bound provides information, it gives the Top the ability to make more informed decisions. A Rigger is not psychic after all. Even a partner who is embracing their dominance cannot be expected to know everything if facts are not being shared.

In the giving and receiving of energy, one form of connection that can arise is that of dominance and submission. The dominant partner asserts control within a scene, or exercises control within a power-based relationship. The submissive partner cedes power within a scene, or surrenders control within a power-based relationship. Dominance is an action, while to be "a Dominant" is a personal identity. The same can be said of someone who chooses to submit or surrender their will (action), or be "a Submissive" (identity).

Not all Dominants play with Submissives, and vice versa. For example, a Dominant might be in a relationship with a Brat, choosing to partner with someone who challenges their dominance, and makes them work harder for the prize. A Submissive might choose to partner with a Hedonist who is excited about binding them and "using" their body, but is more than happy to receive the submission during their play date.

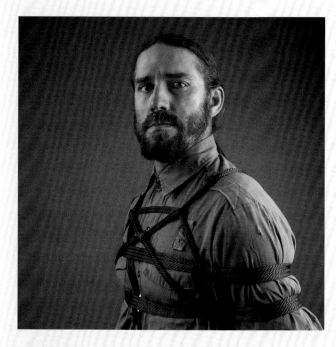

It takes having your own internal power to hand over that power over to someone else.

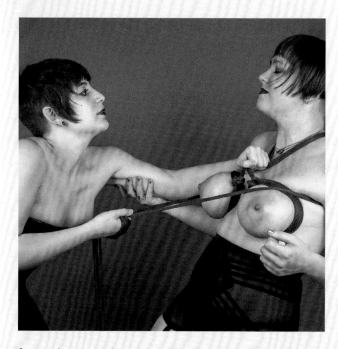

Some people request in advance to have their submission "earned" through struggle.

Asserting dominance has nothing to do with whether you growl at your partner, are sweet to them, or dress in a certain manner. It is certainly not about stepping over anyone's boundaries or limits. In fact, doing so is not dominant in any way—it is rude, mean, and perhaps even abusive. Take care that while you are developing your dominant style, you do so with respect for the gift you have been given. In turn, when submitting, remember that the gift you are giving has value and deserves to be treated as such. The Dominant is being vulnerable as well when giving you their full energy.

There are a number of techniques to consider when adding an element of power exchange to your rope bondage. These include:

Height disparity

The King and I had it right. When someone stands over another person, it has a good chance of affecting the perception of the connection between them. Having your partner kneel or sit can be a great place to start, as can binding your partner into poses like a **Ball Tie** or **Asian-style Hogtie** (as shown in *Shibari You Can Use*). For some individuals, having the Rigger wear a pair of high heels or platform boots can help create this result as well.

Affecting their senses

Blindfolds, hoods and sound-reduction headphones can have someone's focus shift from the world at large to the bondage scene they are in. The touch of your ropes can have more of an impact in doing so. Even the act of binding them so they can only look in a specific direction, and then doing something out of sight, can plant the message that you have more control than they do.

Using your voice

Just as the tone of various musicians and bands have made way for lovers to enjoy each other, having a voice that reflects your dominance can craft a mood as well. A silly voice can set a silly tone. A feral growl can imply that a Bottom will be your prey. Barking commands might get their inner cadet to emerge.

Whispering pornographic ideas can get some folks aroused, but not everyone. In fact, some folks can enter into a trance using the power of silence, or hearing a rhythmic drum beat. Consider for yourself when it is best to talk, and whether exploring quiet might be useful.

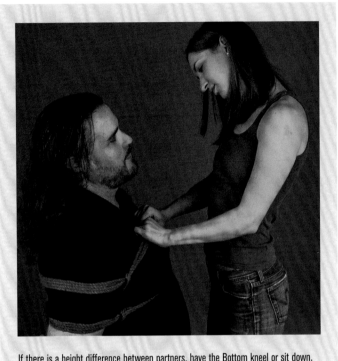

If there is a height difference between partners, have the Bottom kneel or sit down.

Celebrate their experience

When your partner gets turned on, there is a chance for you to get turned on as well. Take a moment mid-scene to pause and see where they are at. If they are reveling in their submission, it may inspire you further into dominance, or simply to be happy for where they are at energetically. If they are feeling powerful in their dominance, it may inspire your own experience of powerful connection, or encourage further surrender. Opening yourself up to feeling their emotions, and letting them feel yours, can help develop the flow of energy between you, and deepen intimacy. This applies whether engaging in dominance and submission or not.

Touch and physicality

Grabbing someone by the hair and pulling them in close. Slowly sliding a firm hand down their exposed body. Seductively running lines of rope over their skin. Using the power of your touch can be a hot way to get people into a space of dominance and submission.

Physical interaction is not just about touch. It can be about weight—resting your feet on them while they are bound. It can involve orders—making them crawl partially tied to go grab the next bundle of rope with their teeth. It can be about dishevelment—removing clothes after they are bound or using their own underwear as a gag or blindfold.

Set an intention

Whatever your intention is, power exchange or otherwise, take a moment before you tie to hold that intent in your mind's eye. In the case of dominance, intentions might include control, ownership, connection, or raw sexual energy. With each piece of the tie, fill the bondage with that intention. By imbuing the ropework with the "why" of your tie, there is a higher likelihood of it being experienced by your partner, as you will be feeling it yourself. Make sure that all parties are on the same "why" and desire for depth before you begin though, lest the passion of one partner be experienced as coercion or manipulation by the other.

Control how the rope comes off

There are many folks who believe that once someone is coming out of rope, the chance for eroticism is over. You are just getting them out of rope, right?

That is not the case. There are just as many steps to untying as there are to getting our partner bound. Unbinding our partner is an excellent chance to get closer to them, emotionally and physically. Sensually touch them as they wiggle free, or firmly pull on each rope you release them. Use the tails of the rope as a tool for brushing against nipples, sweeping across skin, and slowly caressing their flesh. Just when they think you are getting them the rest of the way out, firmly rewrap the lines around their body.

Wrapping your body around your Model can show you are energetically holding onto them as well. Whether they are standing and you are putting your arms around them, or they are seated and you have a leg draped across their body, this sort of contact can plant a subliminal note of control or connection. If you add purpose around how you are dealing with the "finished" rope, it can deepen the control. Are you re-coiling rope as you pin them down, or are you dropping the ropes as they fall while kissing their neck? Is the untying happening at a constant speed, or pausing as you go, catching their breath? Consciousness around untying gives you another place to insert intention.

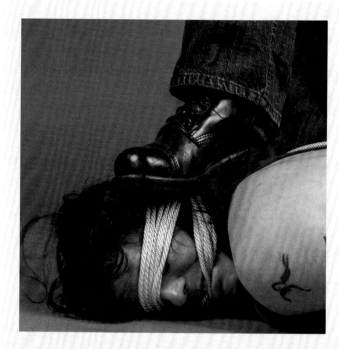

Surrendering power can be hot for some play partners, with the Dominant sitting on the floor in this image, foot gently resting on their play partner.

One of the beautiful things about nawaza (floor bondage with focus and intent), is that we have a chance to be fully in the moment. When we do so, our desires and passionate roles flow forth. We embrace our dominance, submission, sensuality, and interpersonal connection.

If your first time trying out power exchange roles does not go as hoped, try debriefing afterwards. Make sure both partners not only share with compassion, but listen with compassion. When a partner is sharing information, they likely are not intending to be mean. Perhaps the Bottom found the speed of the bondage did not match with your tone of voice. Maybe the Rigger wanted the Model to show their submission by keeping their eyes downcast during the scene. Or, it might be that you both realize you would rather be making art and having hot sex, without these kind of roles involved. There is nothing wrong with any of these. They are all opportunities for learning and modifying your play for next time.

Exercise: Moving Them, Moving You

As part of the physicality of your play, there are two different approaches to how rope goes on the Model's body. The first involves the Model staying still while the rigger walks around them. In doing so, it can feel like a Rigger is stalking their prey, wrapping up a present, or decorating their darling. The second is to have the Rigger stand still, while the Model is turned in circles. This can lead to the Rigger controlling their Model's body, keeping them on their toes.

There are approaches other than moving them or moving you.

A Top can stand behind their Bottom and loop their arms (and rope) around the Bottom. Two Tops can stand on each side of a Bottom and pass the rope back and forth. Rope Bottoms can help a Top tie or untie them, or even put on a self-bondage show while the Top gives them orders from time to time. Whichever route you choose, do so consciously as an active tool for expressing your dominance.

The following exercise explores these two different approaches, using a single 25-30ft (8-10 meter) piece of rope.

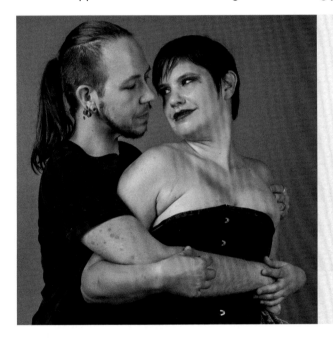

Eye contact

Holding your rope in hand, lock eyes with your partner and connect with them. One form of eye gazing to start with is to have partners gaze left eye to left eye, breathing slowly in time with one another.

1

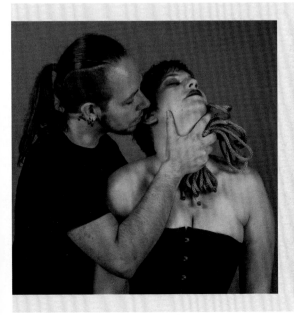 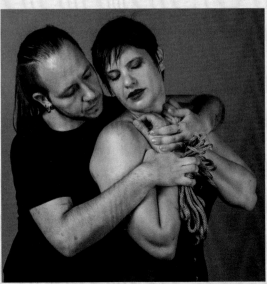

Physical connection

Grab their hair or gently caress their neck, pulling them into the place where you desire them to be standing. Hold their arms and move them into the position you want them to be bound in. This can also be done using verbal orders.

2

Move yourself

Having folded the rope in half, pull the doubled line around their body and create a lark's head in the back. Push your body into theirs. Wrap around their body a second time, walking around them or regularly moving to get your best view or position possible.

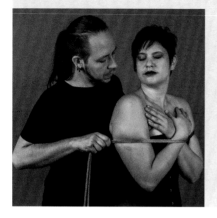 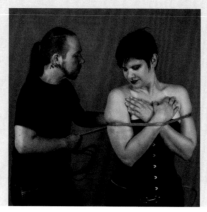 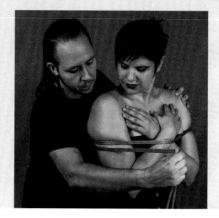

Move them

For the third wrap around their body, slowly turn their body to have their movement do the binding for you. Be careful if your partner is blindfolded, being moved fast, or being moved without having a firm hold on them. It is very easy for a Model to get dizzy, or even fall over. This can become even more of a concern when untying them by having them move, as they spin like a top.

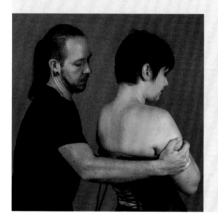 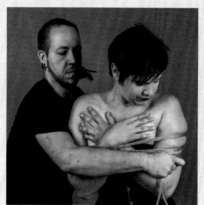 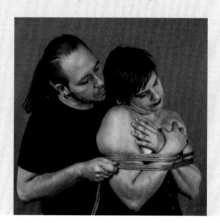

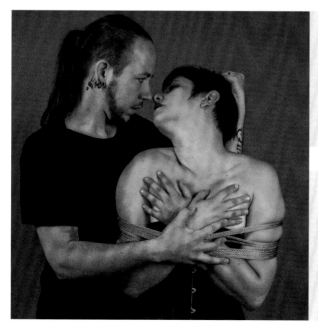

Eye contact

Reconnect with your partner by reestablishing the eye contact used at the beginning of the exercise. If they got dizzy at all, this is another chance to stabilize them against your body, providing for their safety as well.

Whether we have power dynamics actively at play in our rope bondage, the notions of power, consent, movement, and intention are important to consider with any form of bondage play. Power is one of the ingredients that allow us to move from engaging with our rope, to engaging with the person and the moment.

Modified Ties

In the book *Shibari You Can Use*, the **Basic Chest Harness** and **Rope Corset** were included for both restrictive and decorative bondage. In this chapter, we will be looking at ties inspired by those forms.

Adapting our ties to the partners we are playing with shows that we care. We can emulate the works of others, but the models we see in books or pornography are not identical in shape and desire to the person we are together with. They may have more cleavage, less body hair, fewer curves, or have different levels of mobility. Being inspired by the individual form of our lover and altering the tie accordingly shows our Model that we want to play with them specifically, not some generic person.

Part of playing with the person in front of us is keeping the stream of communication with our partner going throughout the scene. A Rigger can look at your body and see where flesh bulges or discolors in ways that look distressing, but only the Bottom can tell a Rigger whether it is actually uncomfortable. Bottoms may like the snugness, or the tie that seems okay is causing tingling, discomfort, nausea, pinching or other unexpected sensations. Let your Rigger know.

Listen to your intuition. If either the Model or Top has a feeling that the tie is not working, consider tying something different. Unrig what was done and have a scene continue after a break or moment of reconnecting. If either of you is not seeming to "click" with rope try something other than rope for this scene like a sexy spanking or good old sex! You can also lovingly say thank you for what you have done so far and finish your encounter.

Have fun playing with your ties, and remember why you are playing in the first place. Modifying your ties might help you craft a roleplaying experience. You can explore gender-bending with feminization (with curves, breasts and hips) or masculinization (with triangular or square torsos and broad shoulders). Try using these ties to manifest gladiators, human ponies, Celtic priestesses or sensual concubines. See where your imagination takes you.

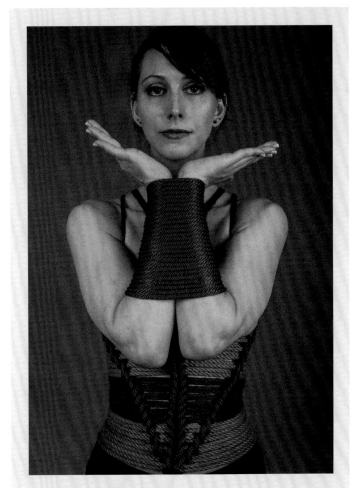

When you see the Fancy Rope Corset from *Shibari You Can Use* where does it inspire you to go next?

Pentacle Harness

This harness features a five-pointed star centered over the heart. The location of the star creates a fantastic opportunity for focusing on the feelings of your heart as you tie this tie, sending that emotional "current" back and forth between you and your partner if you desire. Rope transmits physical vibration, and the same can be said of energy. Together we are weaving our realities with each other. Transmitting our vibrations to one another should only be done with the consent of both parties.

Try combining this tie with breath practices. One way is to breathe in and out as the same time as our partner. Look in each other's eyes and breathe in at the same time. Release at the same time. It also works to breathe in as they release their breath, creating a circuit between you and your partner.

In this tie we are using a 25-35ft (8-11 meter) piece of rope. Stating the intentions suggested in the steps below is optional.

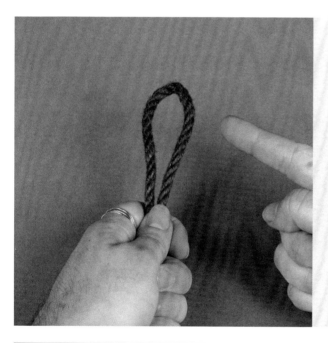

Find the bight

Fold your rope in half. Do whatever sexy or playful look you like, locking eyes with your partner, or blindfold your partner in advance to create even more delight at the end when you unveil your artistic creation.

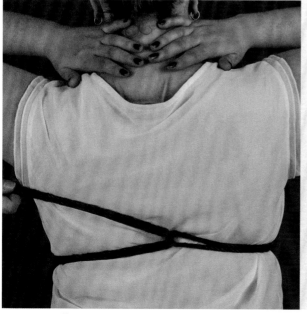

Create lark's head

Wrap your doubled line around the torso just underneath the pectoral mass. Pull the ends through the bight, then pull the ends back in the direction they came from, creating reverse tension on the lines. The lines around the torso should be snug, but not restrictive.

2

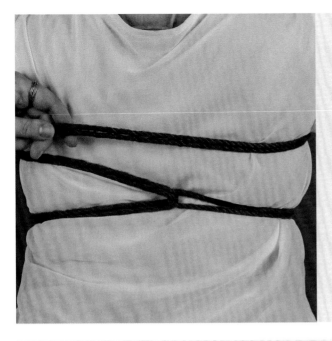

Wrap above the breasts

Continue in the direction determined by the lark's head.

3

Tie off

Pull the ends through your newest created loop/space, then pull back in the direction that you came from, creating reverse tension. Using an overhand knot around all of the chest lines, tie off the back of the harness.

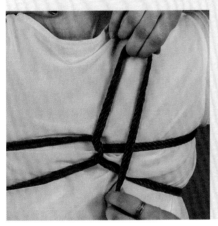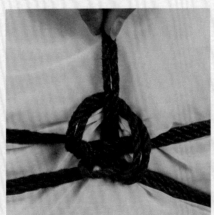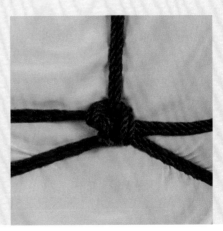

4

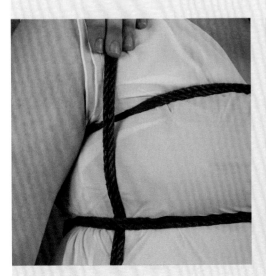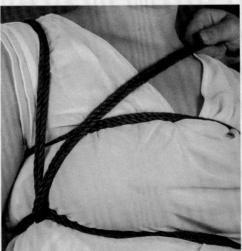

Tuck under and cross body

Bring the rope to the front of the body over the right shoulder. Go underneath the wrap under the breasts on the side nearest the armpit. Snug up slightly and cross over the body, above the breasts, bringing it over the left shoulder.

5

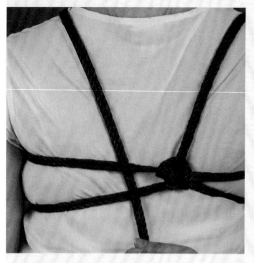
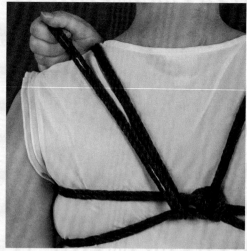

Tuck under and return

Pull the lines underneath all of the torso wraps in the back, near the center knot. Return over the same shoulder, just on the outside of the last shoulder strap.

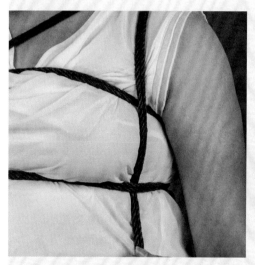
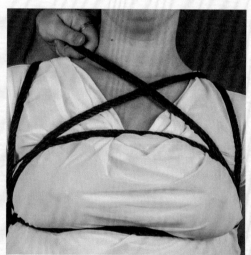

Tuck again and cross body

Go underneath the wrap that is under the breasts near the armpit on the left side of the body. Snug up slightly before crossing over the body, above the breasts, bringing it over the right shoulder.

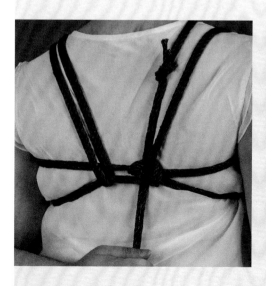
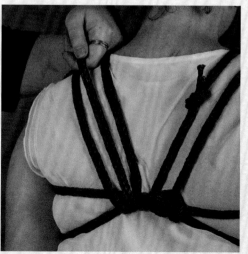

Tuck under and go over other shoulder

Pull your lines underneath all of the torso wraps in the back, near the center knot. Return over the opposite shoulder, between the previous two shoulder straps. **Add rope** (see page 50) if needed.

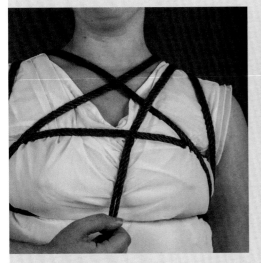
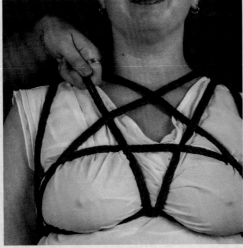

Weave a star

Cross over the first line you encounter, then tuck underneath the upper chest wrap. Go over then under the lower chest wrap. As you come back up, cross over the upper chest wrap, and underneath the last line on that side.

9

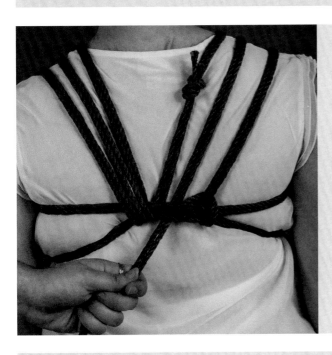

Drop over shoulder and tuck

Return over the shoulder as the center shoulder strap on that side, and tuck underneath all of the chest wraps.

10

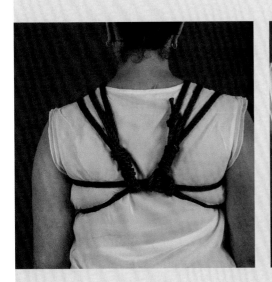
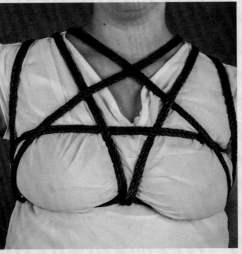

Split lines and tie off

Take the two strands of your rope and split them apart. One line will wrap around all three shoulder straps on the left side before tucking or tying off. The other line will wrap around the shoulder straps on the right side before tucking or tying off. Take a moment while tying off to adjust the distance between the straps to make sure the star falls evenly on the front of the harness.

11

Combining Concepts

With the **Pentacle Harness** in your kinky tool kit, try combining it with other concepts! The image on the cover of the book, for example, combines the tie with a **Rope Corset.** You can take any of the ties in this book, or others (see page 122), and see how they work together.

As you play with these ties, think about all of the different combinations that could take place. Combining ties is one thing, but what about combining our bondage with other types of play. If your partner enjoys spanking, you can bind them in a pair of **Texas Handcuffs,** (see page 36) pull them safely over your lap, and aim at the fleshy parts eager for touch. You can try some of these ideas with your rope:

- Sensory deprivation/control (blindfolds, hoods, earplugs)
- Impact toys (paddles, canes, floggers, whips)
- Impact touch (spanking, slapping, erotic punching)
- Sexual play (oral, anal and vaginal touch/penetration, vibrators, making out, sex toys)
- Fetish play (leather, rubber, high heels, body worship)
- Erotic embarrassment (dirty talking, objectification, furniture role-playing)
- Other forms of bondage (saran wrap, collars, chains, sleep sacks)

Remember as you are exploring these ideas that both parties need to agree to the play. Surprising someone with face slapping could lead to poor responses if it turns out that it is linked to part of their life history. Surprise goes both ways. A Bottom showing up in a beautiful latex catsuit covered in lubrication, inside and out, which might damage some ropes.

Think through how these combinations will interact with the bondage. Low-temperature wax play will leave wax on your rope. Saran wrap can take away those tiny body movements that help some Bottoms endure. Paddles on top of knots can hurt more as they bruise deeper. Wearing a collar can turn tilting your head back into an unplanned form of asphyxiation.

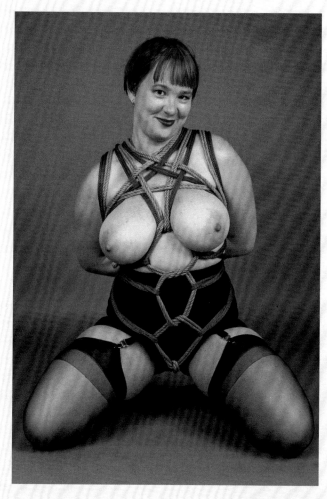

Going over the Pentacle Harness twice can create visually dramatic patterns.

Each and every scene is unique, even if you are doing the same tie you have done many times before. Your play will be an act of teamwork, and that is part of what makes rope bondage such a delight. Don't set formal expectations or comparisons to past scenes. Let this opportunity be the one-of-a-kind experience that it is.

Suspender Harness

Lines that squeeze together at the center of the chest, even on individuals without much tissue there, can create the visual impression of breasts. Such an aesthetic is not desired by everyone, especially those wishing to show a more masculine presentation. This tie is one way to create a more angular design on the chest, painting strong lines and reducing curves.

When working with people with body hair, remember to pull slowly across the skin, or better yet, lay the rope down on the body rather than pulling the rope at all. Make sure not to catch body hair between strands of rope and accidentally pull them out. Some people enjoy using cornstarch on furry bodies in combination with artificial fibers like MFP or nylon, which can aid in smooth sliding, but requires cleanup afterwards.

This tie was executed using 30ft (10 meters) of 8mm jute rope. A larger line was used to be visually proportional to his body shape, rather than the 6mm used elsewhere in this book.

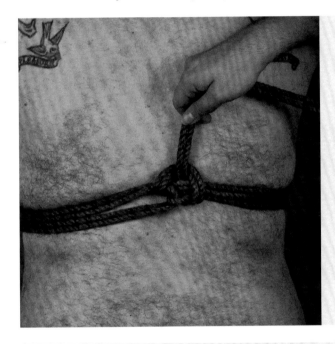

Lay lower chest lines

Follow **steps 1-5 (modified)** from the **Pentacle Harness** (see page 100). As you tie these wraps, keep both sets of wraps below the pectoral mass in this variation.

1-5

Lay upper chest lines

Having tied off the first two wraps, wrap the line around the upper torso. Catch the first (new) wrap, and return in the direction you came from, creating reverse tension. **Add rope** (see page 50) as needed.

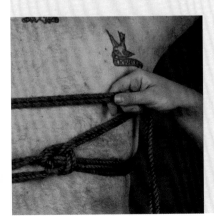
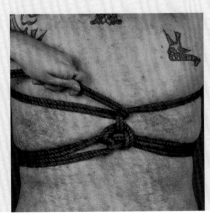
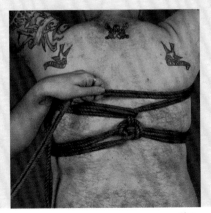

6

Lark's head and tie off

Catch the second (new) wrap, and return in the direction you came from, creating reverse tension. Pull the line up above the upper wraps, letting the tails fall. Take fingers from your open hand, insert them into the triangle, and draw the running ends up creating a half hitch knot.

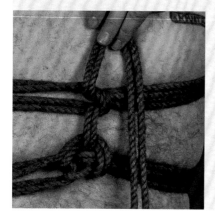
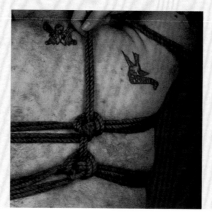
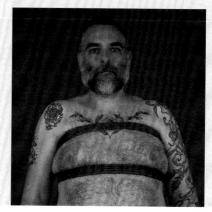

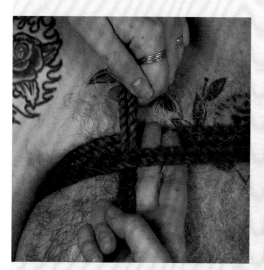
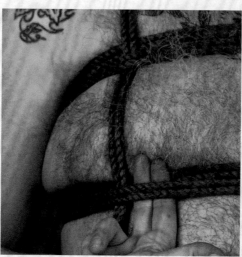

Weave down

Bringing the rope over their shoulder, pass over the first pair of upper chest wraps, and then pass under the second set of upper chest wraps. Pull the rope away from the body as you do so to reduce the chance of rope burn or catching body hair. Laying the rope in a straight line down the body, pass over the first pair of wraps on the lower chest, and then pass under the second set of ropes.

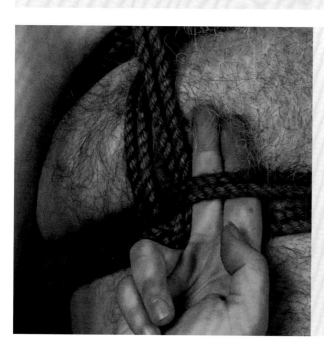

Weave up, part 1

Changing direction, weave over the first wrap you come to, and then under the second wrap. These lines should lay parallel to and touching each other, with the new line closer to the center of the body.

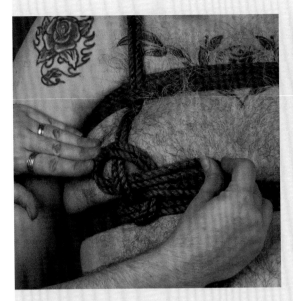
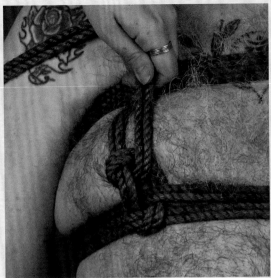

Half hitch knot

Wrap around the line that came down, and bind a half hitch knot around it. Pull down firmly. On his particular body, this is an opportunity for nipple stimulation.

10

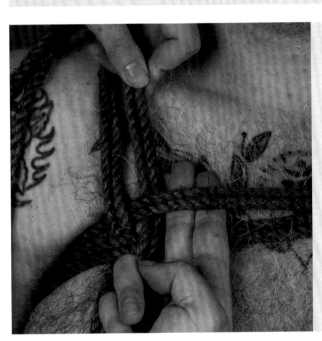

Weave up, part 2

Changing direction, weave over the first wrap you come to and then under the second ropes. These lines should lay parallel to and touching each other, with the new line closer to the center of the body.

11

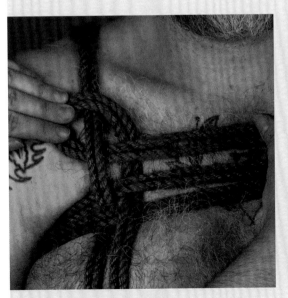
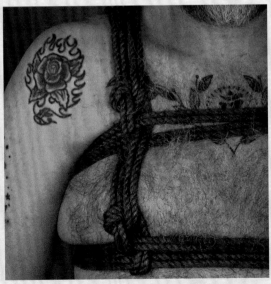

Half hitch knot

Wrap around the line that creates the shoulder strap and bind a half hitch knot around it. Pull down firmly.

12

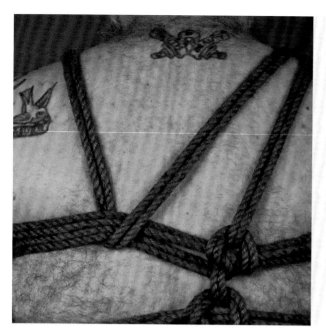

Catch top wraps in back

Bring the rope over the shoulder, crossing to the other side of the back. Lay the line over the upper chest wraps, then come up underneath them before going up over the other shoulder.

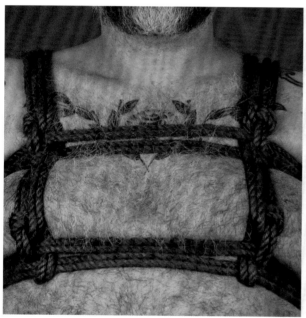

Repeat steps 9-13

As you repeat the steps, make sure to mirror the amount of tension applied to each side of the body to keep the lines as angular as possible. Thus, the lines coming "up" are closer to the center of the body than the lines going "down."

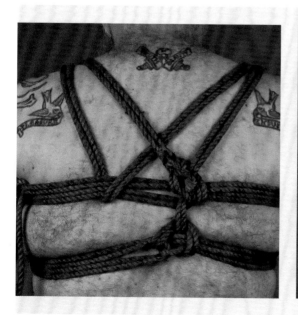

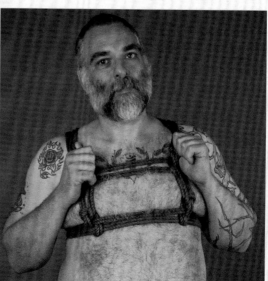

Tie off

Going over the shoulder, cross to the other side of the back and tie off. With additional rope you can create additional detailing with angular lines on the front and back of the body.

Exposure Harness

So many chest harnesses are based off on the idea of lines above and below the breasts, and those lines attached to one and another in some way. But you don't have to be limited in that way. Perhaps your Bottom will be lying on their stomach, and lower chest ropes will be uncomfortable. It could be that they are a mid-chest breather (see page 17). Maybe it is a matter of aesthetics, or you want their torso exposed in general. The Exposure Harness provides an example of how to get your creative juices flowing, with some decorative embellishments (such as the row of Munter hitches shown in this tie) to play with in your future creations.

As the top line will be coming up into the armpit, make sure to check in with your partner about how their arm feels. This is especially true if the line is cinched in or if their arms are pulled behind their back pushing their chest out. They know their body best.

This tie is created using 20-30ft (6-10 meters) of MFP rope.

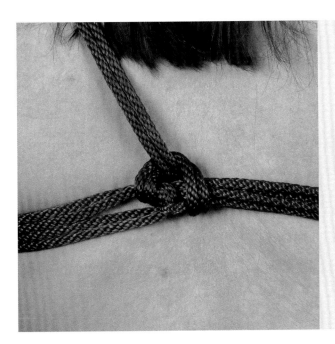

Lay upper chest lines

Follow **steps 1-5 (modified)** from the **Pentacle Harness** (see page 100). As you tie these wraps, keep both sets of wraps above the pectoral mass in this variation.

1-5

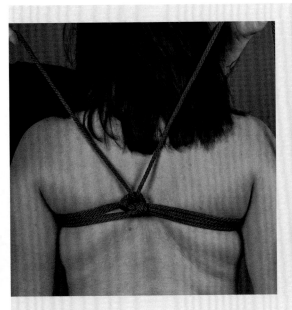
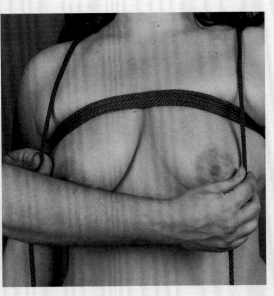

Split lines

Separate the two ropes used to tie the overhand knot, taking one strand over each shoulder.

6

Lock off first strand

Separate the first strand of the four lines on the upper chest. Bring the left rope down, lay the rope across the free strand, and then pull it back up on the outside (closer to the armpit). Cross the line just laid, and then bring the rope down under the chest line on the side closer to the center of the chest. In doing so, you have created a Munter hitch.

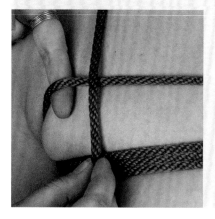 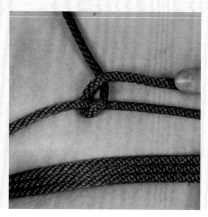 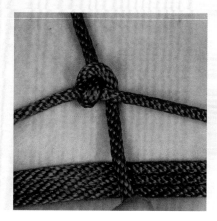

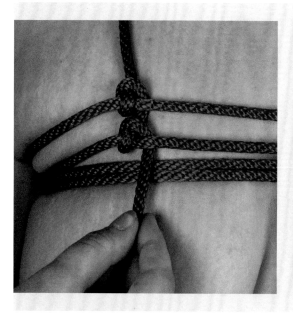 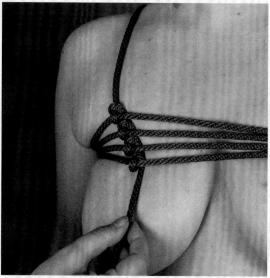

Repeat Munter hitch

Repeat the steps for the Munter hitch to lock off with the next three strands, with the hitches touching, but not overlapping.

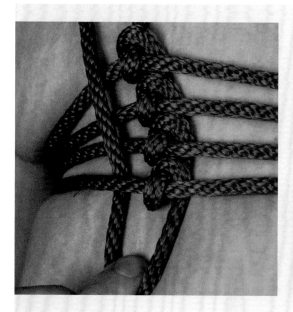 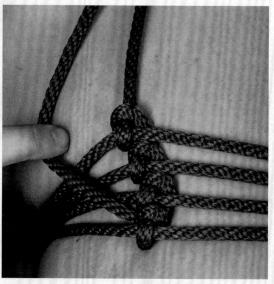

Tuck under bottom line

Tuck the rope underneath the bottom chest line on the side closer to the armpit. As you pull it tight, part of it will seem to disappear behind the decorative lock off details.

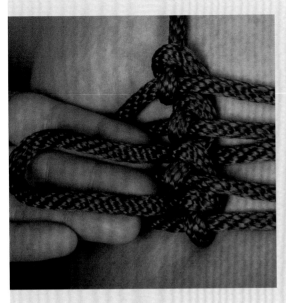
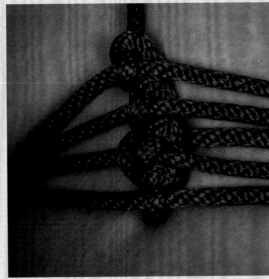

Wrap over then under

Weave over the third chest line from the top, and then pass the rope underneath the lock off details. Emerge on the right side of the decorative details, and pull tight.

10

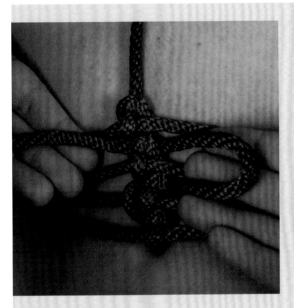
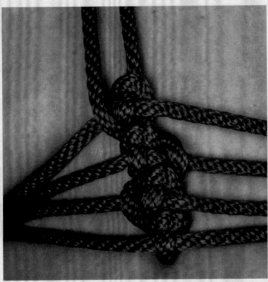

Wrap over then under

Weave over the second chest line from the top, and then pass the rope underneath the lock off details. Emerge on the left side of the decorative details, and pull tight.

11

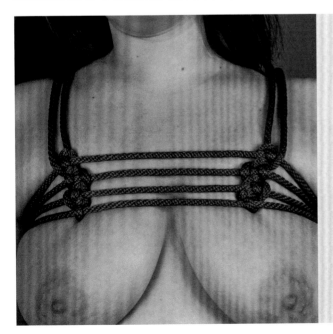

Repeat on the right

Repeat steps 7-11 on the right side of the upper chest, mirroring the work done on the left. Make sure that the Munter hitches are mirroring by following the relationship to the outside of the body (the side closer to the armpit).

12

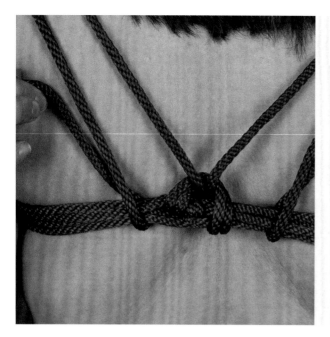

Tuck in back

Bring both lines to the back. Go over the chest wraps, and then under, coming out above the chest wraps on the outside.

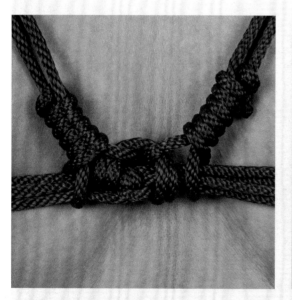

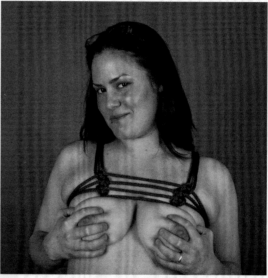

Twist to tie off

Wrap the loose left line around both of the left shoulder straps. Tie off with a knot, or tuck the line between the two shoulder straps and push down. Repeat on the right side.

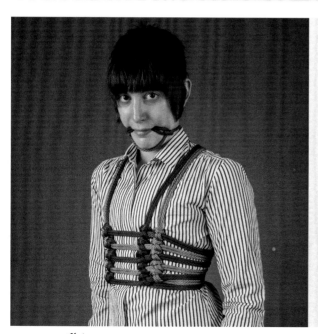

Using the template of the exposure harness, other concepts can be woven. This two-tone version was done by doing three blue wraps and laying one set of Munter hitches down from the shoulders. Having reached the bottom, the lines were brought back and tied off. The teal lines were then wrapped twice around between the blue lines, followed by adding the Munter hitch teal shoulder straps. The lines were brought back and tied off, completing this sleek form.

Speed-Release Corset

When playing, sometimes I like the drama of a long, involved tie that comes off very quickly. This is the case with this fun piece of ropework.

Remember to check in with your Model from time to time and see how they are doing, as creation of the decorated version of this tie can take a while. This affects both their breathing capacity and your interpersonal connections. Pause every once in a while to kiss their body or smack them on the ass. Share with them how beautiful, sexy or delightful they look. Blindfold them and let them sink into the sensation of the rope or the music you have chosen to play in the background. Remind them you are not so absorbed in the technical aspects of tying that you have forgotten there is a person in all of that rope!

This specific corset was achieved using a 28 inch (70cm) cane and five 25-30ft (8-10 meter) pieces of jute.

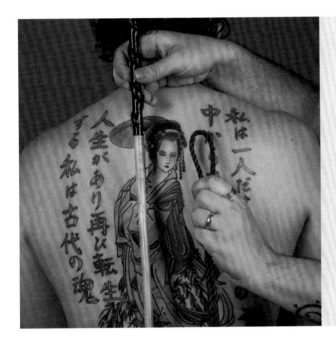

Acquire a cane

Though any smooth stick will do, I like the charm of using a rattan cane. It will allow the "spine" of the corset to double as a tool for other erotic encounters. The cane should be smooth and less than an inch thick (2.5 cm). The length will depend on what you are corseting. For a waist-cincher, 16 inches (40 cm) is plenty on most bodies. For a hip to upper chest corset, you will need to adjust the length accordingly.

1

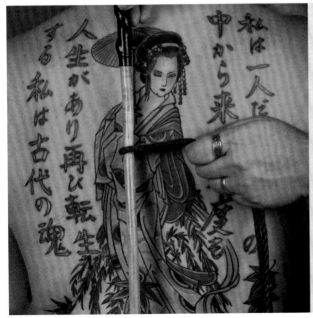

Slide bight over cane

Fold the rope in half, and slide the cane into the center point.

2

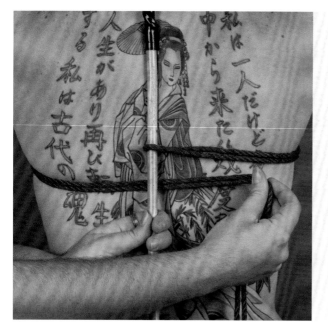

Wrap around and pass under

Holding the cane in place centered over the spine (or reverse the tie with the cane centered in front), wrap around the torso, just above the chest. Pas under the cane by sliding the doubled rope just beneath where you began the tie.

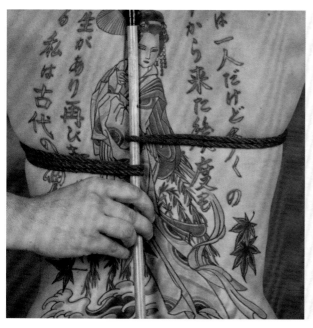

Reverse direction

Holding the cane in place, wrap around the torso in the opposite direction, directly under the first wrap. This second line will wrap directly below the first one, also above the chest.

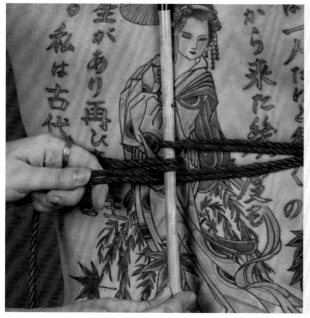

Pass under cane

Slide the doubled rope under the cane, just beneath where the last rope passed around the cane.

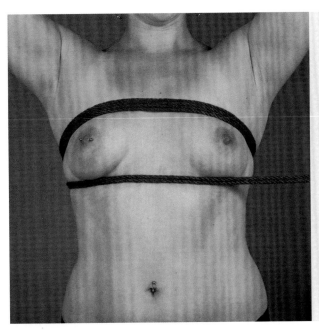

Reverse direction

Holding the cane in place, wrap around the torso in the opposite direction, with lines from here forward wrapping underneath the chest.

6

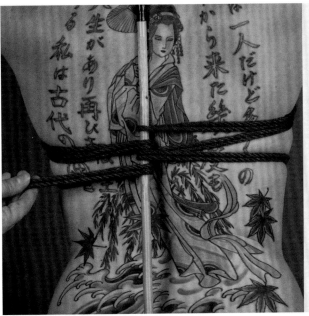

Repeat steps 5 and 6 until you reach the bottom

Wrap just below the last line each time as you continue down the torso. Make sure to keep tension even with each wrap and straighten the cane to keep it centered. It is important that you change directions each time, rather than wrapping entirely around the body by going in a single direct at any point. If you do so, the corset will not, in fact, be speed-release any more.

7

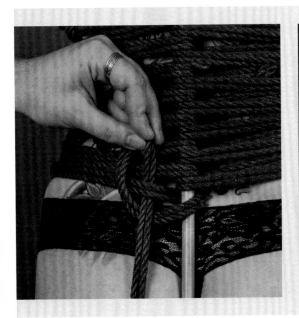

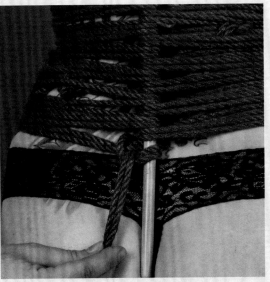

Tie off

When you reach the end of your corset, tuck the ropes under the cane one last time. Reverse the direction, and tie a half hitch knot on the side you just came from.

8

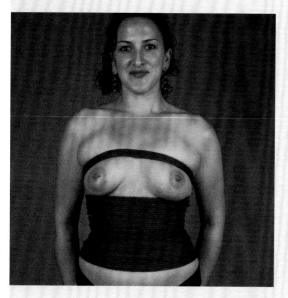 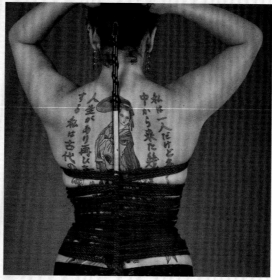

Tuck the rope ends away

At this point, the rope corset is finished, unless you choose to decorate.

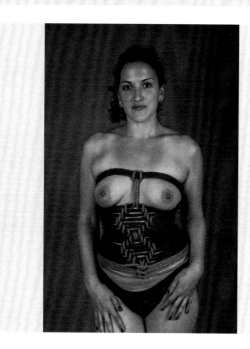

(optional) Decorate

Have fun adding decorative details to the front of the corset. You can lay a second spine in the front, create rows, make patterns, or use multiple colors. With each rope that you add, the corset will get tighter. Check in with your partner regularly to see how they are doing.

But wait, didn't we say it was speed release? Well, if that's the case, we need to see how fast it comes off!

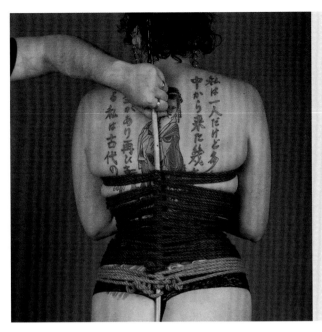

To open the corset...

Grab hold of the top of the cane

Make sure you have a firm grip.

1

Pull upwards

As you pull up slowly on the rod, watch the corset fall away! Moving from being tightly bound to being instantly released can create a profound sense of vulnerability due to the intense change in sensation, so be aware that some Models may have difficulties with the quick transition.

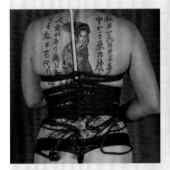 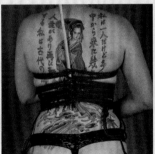 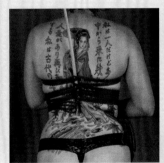 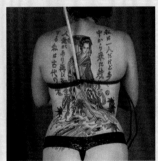

2

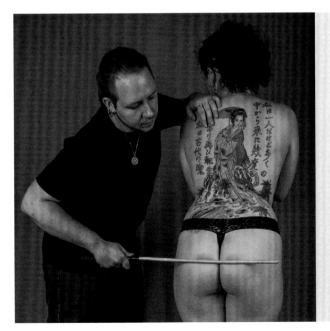

(optional) Follow through with a cane stroke!

This can transition into an erotic caning scene if the Model is a fan of such antics. Moving from being tightly bound to being instantly released can create a profound sense of vulnerability due to the intense change in sensation, so beware that some Models may have difficulties with the quick transition.

Canes can be an intense tool to use. They can leave heavy marks when landing hard blows and the tip of the cane travels quicker than the rest of it (and more painfully). Begin gently, and build up having learned how to use the tool, and having explored your partner's desires.

3

Exercise: Developing Mindfulness

In our erotic lives, most of us have stories rolling around in our heads. Examples of these stories include:

- What "normal" sex is supposed to look like.
- What our family/friends/community would think if they knew we were doing bondage.
- How our play compares to scenes with past lovers (either our own, or our partner's past lovers).
- How our play today compares to our past scenes with this play partner.
- What our partner is thinking about us right now.
- What this sort of play means about us as people.

Most of these stories have nothing to do with what is going on in the moment. Our story to ourselves that our partner thinks we don't look beautiful in this tie most likely is not what our partner is actually thinking. Having these stories in the forefront of our mind means we are not focused on the bondage play that we are actually doing right now. In reality, we are cheating ourselves out of the greatness we could be experiencing.

If we are not present in the moment, we are also not fully present for our partner. That does not make us bad people. It means that we, like most people on the planet, have an opportunity to develop mindfulness in our erotic explorations with one another. Be patient with yourself as you develop this practice. After all, mindfulness is considered a practice because it takes practice.

When your attention slips away while following any of these steps, be kind to yourself as you bring your attention back to the step. In the first attempt at this exercise, you may only be able to hold each step for a few moments. Through repetition of these exercises, your capacity for returning to mindfulness will increase.

Notice the rope

As you pick up the first piece of rope, feel the weight of the rope. How heavy is it? What is the texture in your hand? What color is the rope? What is the smell? How wide are the strands under your fingertips as you slowly wrap the lines around your partner?

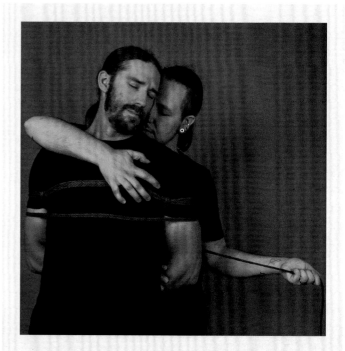

As you begin building mindfulness, start by noticing your rope.

As you are being bound with the first piece of rope, feel the weight of the rope on your skin. What is the texture of it as it glides along over your bare skin, as compared to when it passes over any clothing you may be wearing? What color is the rope? What is the smell? How wide are the strands as they dance across your flesh?

Bring a quality of awareness to what is happening and experiencing now, here, in this moment. There is no set agenda, just now.

As you bind, simply be aware what you are noticing about the rope and the binding that is happening at this time.

Notice your partner

Move your focus from the rope to the person you are doing bondage with. What does their skin feel like? What is the temperature of their body, the texture of their flesh? How are they responding to the scene at this time?

Is the Top breathing heavier as they snug the rope tighter? Is the Bottom moaning slightly as the tips of the jute are dragged across their nipples? By developing an awareness of these responses of our partner, mindfulness can become a powerful tool for erotic charge.

This step is not about trying to illicit a specific response from our partner. When we focus on our own ideas of "if I do this to them, they will do this response," we have left the moment we are in. That type of thinking is telling a story about the future. When we focus on our story, we are no longer bringing our full awareness to the moment. We end up having a scene with our own internal story, rather than having an experience with our partner.

Having this internal scene makes us profoundly human. Humans do this throughout their days, and throughout their lives. Breathe, try again. Move your focus to your partner. Breathe deep, and truly notice them in this moment, in this place and time.

Appreciate their joy

"Compersion" is the experience of feeling pleasure when a loved one feels pleasure. This empathetic state is sometimes referred to as "the opposite of jealousy." Finding its roots in the open relationship community, the original form referred to one person finding joy in the other person experiencing joy with another lover or partner. But the same concept can apply within a single scene and partnership.

Sometimes in bondage scenes, if our partner is enjoying a specific moment more than we are, a possibility for resentment or envy can arise. Instead of begrudging the delight of our partner, we are open to tap into the notion of mudita (a Buddhist term for sympathetic joy), and the inner spring of infinite joy. The more we are rooted in our own delights, the easier it is to delight in the joys of others, and have their joy reflect back our own core joy.

This form of sympathetic or vicarious joy can be accessed by seeing the smile on a partner's face. Hearing them gasp or moan. Feeling the shiver of their body against ours. Listening to their words of appreciation.

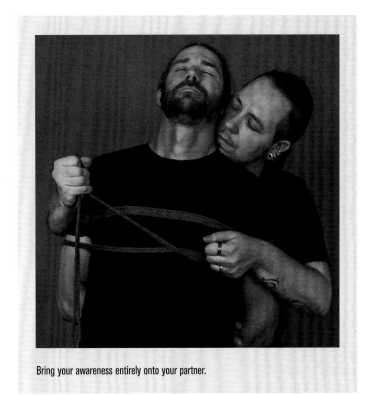

Bring your awareness entirely onto your partner.

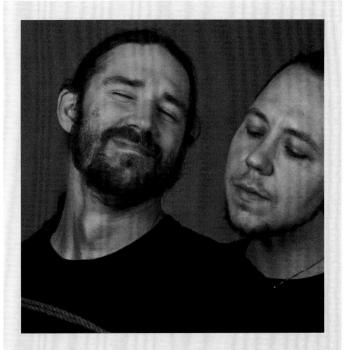

Building compersion and empathy can bring you closer to one another.

Notice the expressions of joy, passion or delight they are experiencing during the scene. Bear witness to it. This form of mindfulness in their joy is about transforming this moment of being present into the next moment of being present.

What is making your partner joyous? What joy can you find in their joy? This is not about sacrificing your own comfort or joy in exchange for theirs. This is about experiencing their joy. Experiencing them in their hotness. In their delight. In their laughter. In their erotic fervor.

Take profound interest in them, and appreciate the gift they are sharing with you.

Be here, now

Mindfulness in bondage is about doing bondage. It is not about looking around a public dungeon to see what other cool scenes are happening. It is not about worrying whether you will be a good enough Rigger or Model. It is about being here, now. This is why doing all of your preparation as both a Model and Rigger is so important, so you have the ability to enter into a place of mindfulness in bondage, if only for a moment. Make sure everyone is safe... but be here, now.

When coiling rope... coil rope.

When you are using rope... use rope.

When tying your partner... tie your partner.

When being bound by your lover... be bound by your lover.

Be here, now.

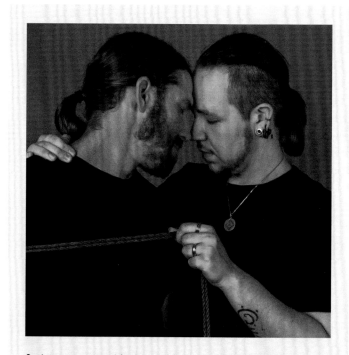

Coming to rope events might give you a chance to connect with someone new.

Moving Forward

With chest harnesses and facial bondage, cuffs and crotch ropes, corsets and hand ties, and many ideas on connecting with our partner... where do we go from here? In this chapter we will look at where to read more, get supplies, learn more and meet others through the rope bondage communities. Though this is *More Shibari You Can Use*, there are even MORE resources out there for you to explore!

You can also consider this chapter a form of aftercare for you, the reader. Aftercare is a tool for transitioning out of a rope scene and back into the world at large. Some people like to curl up in a warm blanket to eat a snack. It may be taking time to coil rope while eye-gazing with your lover. Perhaps your aftercare is some sensual kissing and sharing your favorite moments from your time together. There are even folks who like to spend some time alone "grounding" back into reality after they "flew."

Both Tops and Bottoms will want some form of aftercare, even if it is drinking some water and checking in with a friend days later to see how you are doing after the fact. Without some form of aftercare, it can lead to something called "Sub Drop" or "Top Drop"—a feeling of malaise, depression or even physical illness. Make sure everyone gets their needs met post-scene.

Right after a scene you may still be in an altered state of consciousness from that energetic high. It is not a good time to give critical feedback about the scene. A few hours or days later, take time to see if your partner is available to talk to give them information about what you thought was awesome about the scene as well as what could be improved on. This can help both partners learn, grow and evolve. This is much more useful, and connecting, than blaming our partners or being negative.

Part of learning, growing and evolving is doing so between scenes. So let's look at those additional resources, shall we?

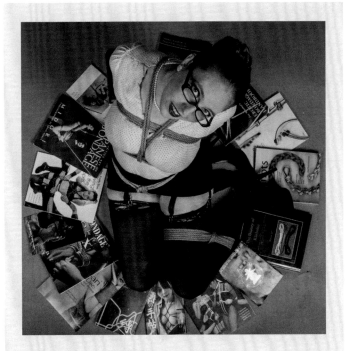

Don't let your learning stop here—keep getting inspired!

Books

This series of bondage books is not the only option available on the market. There are some other books out there that are worth taking a look at. Some are more analytical than others, and each will appeal to different people. Flip through them and decide for yourself, or see the more detailed descriptions of some of these in *Shibari You Can Use*. New projects are being released all the time.

Instructional books:

- *Back on the Ropes* by Two Knotty Boys
- *The Book of Five Rings for Rope Arts, Volumes 1 and 2* by Arisue Go
- *Complete Shibari Volume 1: Land* by Douglas Kent
- *Das Bondage-Handbuch: Anleitung zum erotischen Fesseln* by Matthias Grimme
- *The Erotic Bondage Handbook* by Jay Wiseman
- *The Essence of Shibari* by Shin Nawakiri
- *Kinbaku Mind and Techniques, Volumes 1 and 2* by Arisue Go
- *Rope Bondage: Precision and Persuasion with Rope* by Scott Smith
- *Rope for Sex: Volume 1* by Chanta Rose
- *The Seductive Art of Japanese Bondage* by Midori
- *Shibari: The Art of Japanese Bondage* by Master "K"
- *Shibari You Can Use: Japanese Rope Bondage and Erotic Macramé* by Lee Harrington
- *Showing You the Ropes* by Two Knotty Boys
- *The Toybag Guide to Basic Rope Bondage* by Jay Wiseman

Theory and history books:

- *The Beauty of Kinbaku* by Master "K"
- *The Little Guide to Getting Tied Up* by Evie Vane
- *Rope, Bondage and Power* edited by Lee Harrington and Robert Ruebel

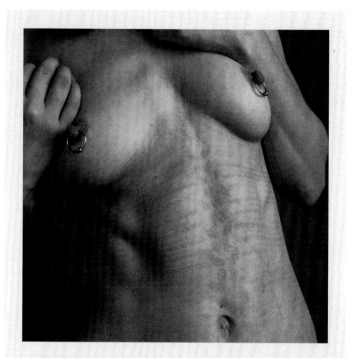

Some people are turned on by rope marks, feeling like they have been "marked" by their partner or made into works of art.

Art books:

- *Bound: Shibari Style Impressions* by David Lawrence
- *Kinky Bondage Obsession: The Best of Bondage Café* by Jim Weathers
- *L.A. Bondage* by David Naz
- *Male Bondage: Art Deserves a Witness* by Van Darkholme
- *Pleasure in the Fall* by Minako Ogawa, a.k.a. Daraku
- *ReBound: Shibari Style Impressions* by David Lawrence
- *Strictly Bondage* by Victor Lightworship

Buying Rope

Nowadays there are numerous options for where to purchase rope. You can also choose to go to your local hardware or sailing supply shop, but the more exotic ropes (or finished ropes that have had all of the splinters removed) will not be available. Listed here are links to some of the erotic rope retailers that are producing beautiful product at the time of publication. Further details on what some of these vendors are known for are available in *Shibari You Can Use*.

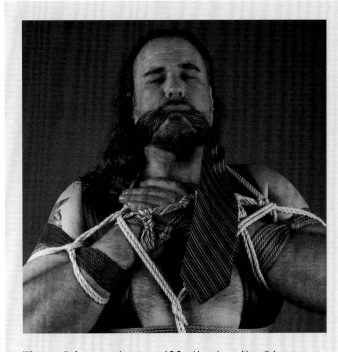

Who says all of your ropes have to match? Consider going multi-media!

- www.RopeExtremes.com
- www.BindMe.nl
- www.AiNawa.com
- www.AjaRope.com
- www.BastardRopes.com
- www.BossBondage.com
- www.DeGiottoRope.com
- www.ErinHoudini.com
- www.Esinem.com
- www.Garrs-Ropes.com
- www.JadeRope.com
- www.Jakara-Rope.co.uk
- www.Jugoya.com
- www.KinkyRopes.com
- www.KnotKnormal.com
- www.KnottyKink.com
- www.MauiKink.com
- www.M0coJute.com
- www.Nawa.tv/rope
- www.RainbowRope.com
- www.RenaissanceRope.com
- www.RopeSpace.com
- www.Serenity-Bound.com
- www.TwistedMonk.com
- www.VenusRopes.com
- www.VintageRope.com
- www.WitherAndDye.com

Supporting rope vendors who are into bondage themselves helps build a continued web of resources for kink enthusiasts. You might also choose to treat your own rope or learn to make rope with your own hands.

Rope Community and Culture

Beyond the books, there is an international flesh-and-blood rope bondage community that has evolved in recent years. From fetish balls to practice sessions, private classes to massive conferences, the ways people into rope are exploring with each other are truly diverse.

Just as the reasons we want to do rope are personal, so it is with getting involved in the rope community. Some want to come because it is a chance to shop, learn skills, or meet experts in the craft. Others long for a space where they can live out a fetish fantasy in person, take in astounding sights and make memories to last a lifetime. You might be coming out to find compatible partners, or to find friends you don't have to explain your passions to. Or maybe you have thin walls and would like a place you can moan as loud as you like.

Knowing your reasons for wanting to get involved in the rope community will help you choose events that will best suit your needs, as well as keep your intentions clear as you move forward. You can also choose not to join a community, playing at home with just this book for inspiration. The choice is up to you.

Gatherings of bondage people come in a wide variety of experiences:

Online

For many, exploring online is a great way to find information, get inspired, and make friends.

Social media sites for kinky people are continuing to pop up. Some are focused on hooking up with play partners. If that appeals to you, look for websites that ask you during sign-up what kinds of play partners and specific activities you are looking for. Others are focused on education, with articles and essays. They might be about sharing art, or looking for in-person local groups (serving more as a local directory, with an associated discussion group).

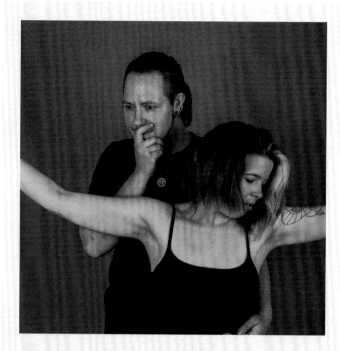

Not sure what to do next? Try looking into some online resources as a start.

Some of these social media sites that include broader connections beyond hooking up include:

- DarkSide.se
- FetLife.com
- FetishMen.net
- KinkCulture.com
- Recon.com

On the site FetLife.com, there are thousands of discussion groups, including a large number that are specifically about rope bondage. The two I recommend as starting points are "Shibari" (group 195) and "Adult Rope Art" (group 2816). The Adult Rope Art group is a continuation of the group founded in the late '90s by Jimi Tatu, and is full of links and resources for exploring not only rope bondage, but the rope bondage community as well.

To find kink events, from munches/get-together events to fetish balls and weeklong retreats, there are also sites online that focus on connecting people in-person:

- DrkDesyre.com
- FetLife.com
- FindAMunch.com
- Leatherati.com
- TheBDSMEventsPage.com

As you are exploring the online world, remember to take care of yourself and your own personal security. Do not post your address, phone number, legal name, or other personal details where others can use them for their own purposes. Think twice before putting up images of yourself—once something is on the internet, it might just stay on the internet. Many people create screen names or "scene names" to help them navigate online. You may want to consider whether it is a name you are okay being referred to by online, and perhaps also saying out loud when you go to your first in-person gathering. And remember—you don't need an online profile to have fun in the community.

If you are new to exploring the kink or rope communities online or in person, consider getting a copy of *Playing Well With Others: Your Guide to Discovering, Exploring and Navigating the BDSM, Kink and Leather Communities* by Lee Harrington and Mollena Williams. It is full of resources on planning in advance, navigating events, meeting new people, and figuring out how to integrate your new kinky life into your life at large.

Not all online exploration is about meeting people. Sometimes it is about the hot porn! There are lots of bondage websites that you can go get turned on by. The cool thing about these sites is now that you have some rope-tying knowhow, you can start replicating a few of those ties in your own bedroom. The problem? Some of the ties you will see are not practical or even possible for most Models or Riggers. The moments where Models express a need to get untied get edited out of the final footage, just like when Models fart. Remember to play in person with the person in front of you, not the porn ideals. Models fart, and so do Riggers.

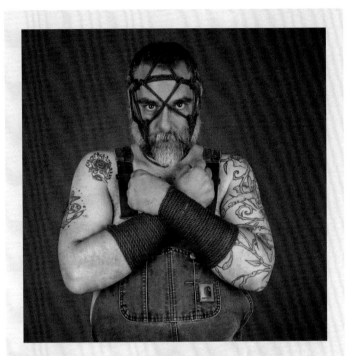

Online you will find people into rope for many reasons—don't assume you know their personal passions or story.

You can also look for tutorials online that pick up where this book leaves off. Check out some of these free tutorials and educational resources:

- www.BastardRopes.com
- www.BeKnotty.com
- www.JapaneseRopeArt.com
- www.JapanBondage.tv
- www.Kikkou.com
- www.KinkyClover.com
- www.MassachusettsBondage.com
- www.My-Knots.blogspot.com
- www.NaturallyTwisted.co
- www.Nawapedia.com
- www.RemedialRopes.com
- www.RopeFashions.com
- www.Rope-Topia.com
- www.Shibari-By.com
- www.TwistedMonk.com
- www.TwoKnottyBoys.com

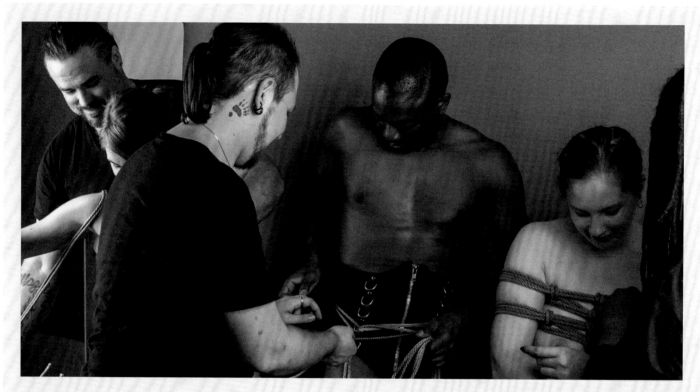

The rope community is a place where rope enthusiasts can connect with other rope enthusiasts.

Munches

Munches are social gatherings, often at public restaurants, cafés or bars, where people get together and talk. You show up in your street clothes, and have conversations. Munches are a great way to meet new people, find out where the local parties are, and get resources. You usually shouldn't bring a big bag of rope with you for playing unless you have talked to the organizer and know that is more of a practice session event (though a few pieces of rope don't take up much room if they are hidden in your bag). Get ready to make friends, generate contacts, and enjoy conversations.

Practice sessions

Sometimes referred to as "Rope Bites" or "Rope Bights," practice sessions are a chance to try out what you know and learn a few new tricks. Bring your rope, bring a partner (though pairing for practice is usually available for Tops or Bottoms, and some people practice self-bondage as well), and let the ropes fly! This is a chance to try out new things, perfect what you already know, and share something with others. After all, having read this book, you already have quite a few things to pass on. You might even meet a new play partner and see how they interact with others before you agree to play with them.

Educational experiences

Learning comes in a lot of shapes and styles in the rope community. This is great, because there is always a chance to learn something new. It is not culturally appropriate to ask people to show you something when they are in the middle of a scene (even if it is at a public party)—so these different educational experiences provide chances to pick up more information.

Classes are the most common form of education available. They range in size from three people in an intimate class to 150 or more (yes, really) being taught at once. Some are taught by internationally-known instructors, or by novice community members who have something to share. Some are held at sex shops, while others are at private homes or university student centers. Find out a few things in advance:

- Who is hosting the event?
- How large is it?
- What is the fee for attending?
- What should you bring?
- Is it for couples only?
- Are there any skill prerequisites for attending?

In some cases, the class is part of a series, and you are expected to sign up for all of the classes in the course. Others are full-weekend experiences, limited to a handful of students, with parties and meals included. Most are stand-alone learning opportunities.

Not everyone is suited to classes, no matter how large or small. They may learn more through mentorship or one-on-one instruction. By joining a rope community, you may be able to find someone who can give you tips and tricks, show you how to do a tie from the basics on up, or learn advanced techniques. Bottoms can find another Bottom to mentor them in how to take rope, negotiate their needs, and explore their headspace.

Learning formally from a mentor, or a private instructor, means you are learning "their" way of doing rope. Some teachers are part of formal systems that have been passed down from teacher to student over and

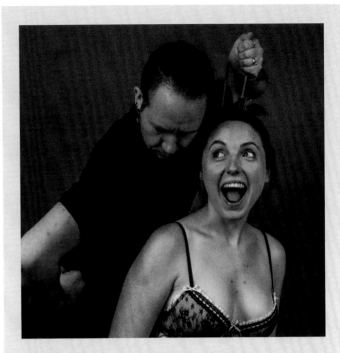

At educational events, practice sessions, and munches, remember to have a good time.

over again. Even though students will make the style their own, the influence of their instructors will often show. Other mentors and teachers have skills that they evolved on their own, and bring their unique excellence to the table.

No two instructors have the same approach to teaching or style of rope. Some are more skilled in how to teach ties step-by-step, and others prefer to have you watch their demonstrations and ask questions afterwards. Find out how a rope teacher shares their bondage techniques, and see if it will work for you.

You can also learn by going to parties and seeing how other people play. The rope community is often very friendly to people who, in the food or social area of a party, ask questions about what someone was doing in their scene. You might just end up learning how to tie a strap-on harness in the middle of the kitchen!

Performance events

From fetish clubs to mainstream performance groups like Cirque du Soleil, bondage has become a prolific tool for erotic entertainment. Some events specialize in the spectacular, with skilled artisans throwing bodies up in the air to flip around in perfect choreography. Others are intimate gatherings, where the patrons can see the ecstasy and agony of the writhing Model on stage.

There are mega-events with a hundred performers and ones with only one show during the course of the night. Local bars might open up their stage to players who want to go-go dance in decorative bondage for all to see. And sometimes, what you thought was a show was actually a handful of party-goers simply enjoying themselves.

Find out in advance what to wear. Some bondage performance and fetish balls events have dress codes, especially if you paid a large ticket price. This is because the producers are trying to create a consensually constructed fantasy experience, where you can be part of the dream. Not being part of that vision can lead to feeling like a "glitch in the Matrix."

Rope and BDSM Parties

Public parties might take place at a swingers or BDSM venue, being advertised online or perhaps posting fliers at a local dance club. They often have an entry fee, and some will include dress codes. Private parties might be part of a larger organization gathering, comprised of folks the organizers know in person (such as from their local munch), or be for only the closest of friends. A party might be for all forms of BDSM play, rope only, be centered on a specific fantasy, be fetish focused, or be a chance for people to take erotic photos. Find out the rules of the party, and what activities and atmosphere might be expected there.

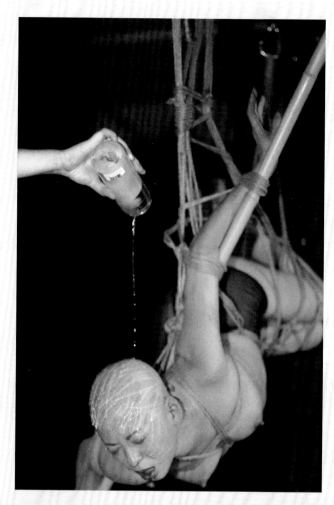

At performance events, you may see a variety of beautiful or extreme rope bondage artistry.

At parties you get to choose how you participate, whether you play in the dungeon with a new play partner, your established partner, or watch other people's scene before going home to play in your own intimate one-on-one space. Coming out to make friends or just watch is also a completely valid option. Come on out whether you are single, partnered, or in an open relationship of some sort. In the vast majority of cases, are all welcome.

Conferences

Rope bondage conferences have sprung up around the globe. Indoor and outdoor, hotel-based and at private venues, each varies in size and style. They might be education-only, or a combination of shopping, classes, parties, contests, performances, and socials where you can get to know other rope enthusiasts.

At BDSM, kink, pornography, and fetish conferences, there might also be a "rope track" or individual rope classes where an interest in erotic restraint brings certain attendees together. You will meet people who have been in the community for 10 years but are just now exploring rope, as well as passionate newcomers who are rope obsessed and have tons to share. Since these more diversified events appeal to a broader demographic, not everyone you meet will be into rope bondage, but everyone will be sharing that they have erotic interests outside of the mainstream norm.

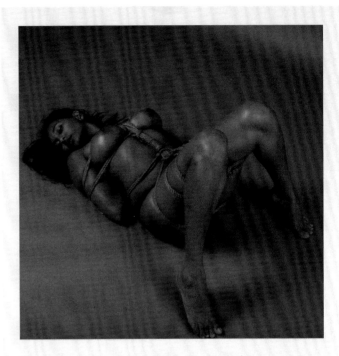

Coming to rope events might give you a chance to connect with someone new.

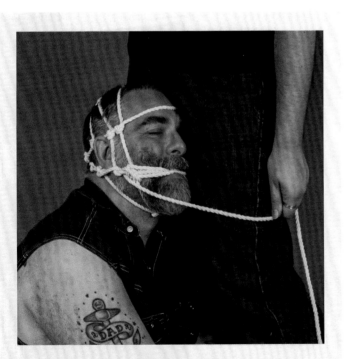

Some people come to the rope community to explore being their authentic selves.

Go Forth and Connect!

That's it? Nope, not at all. Now, it is your turn to take all of this information and make it your own. Practice the ties and exercises in this book, and then begin to combine and craft them into something that works perfectly for who you are, who your play partner is... and who you are together. Find the unexpected joys, and check your assumptions. Treat each other with respect as you dive into your desires.

It is delicious to enjoy rope bondage, but there is so much more to this art form and hot play than the technical skills. You have the tools in hand now to play, have fun, and also create magic.

Breathe deep. Connect with yourself and your desires. Breathe deep once more. Connect with your partner and their desires. Breathe deep... and remember why YOU are here, rope in hand.

Have fun, live life, and enjoy the intimacy and connection of bondage!

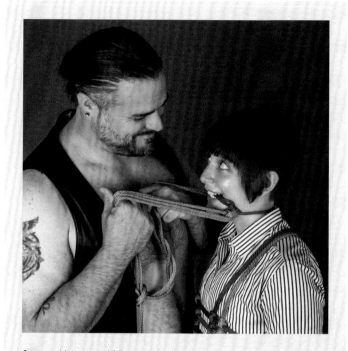

Connect with intent, and follow your own bliss.

Acknowledgements

Three years in production, *More Shibari You Can Use,* has been quite the ride! Friends and fans alike have been asking me for the past six years when it would come to light. Well, here we are, in full beautiful color with a rocking crew having helped make it happen.

Though I originally considered having *More Shibari* be a straight-up bondage manual like the first book in the series, after my book *Sacred Kink: The Eightfold Paths of BDSM* came out, I knew I couldn't have a book without the "why" of bondage included after spending so much time diving into where altered states of consciousness and kinky sex overlap. In *Rope, Bondage and Power* I was honored to edit 20 authors' work as to the "whys" of their own rope journeys—but there was nothing out there to help people make those moments of connection and magic happen for themselves. And one day Aiden Fyre asked me about making such a book happen as a bridge between these two books and the first bondage book, a conversation I am grateful for years later. The new vision was born—to combine "Westernized" Shibari with the connection we all deserve.

When it was decided this project needed to come out, I was honored to be able to pair up with the fantastic RiggerJay. We spent many long days in overheated spaces pouring out our vision and soul, and I am blessed to have had such an amazing adventure mate not only for this book, but also to the revision of the first *Shibari* book. It has been delightful seeing him grow over the years as both a Rigger and a photographic artist, and I am honored to call him a friend as well.

We had an amazing crew of Models to work with— Models of all shapes, sizes, ethnic backgrounds and orientations who were game to rock up and put some diversity into the world of bondage instruction and erotica. Our amazing crew for this book were Amy Morgan, Ay, Ayem Willing, Barracudabite, BendYogaGirl, Calico, Deanna Cannonball, Ginger Baker, Jena, Jester35, Just Derek, Klawdya Rothschild, Knave Karina, Lily Ligotage, Lily Swan, Mecha Kate, Miss Seraph, Mollena Williams, Murphy Blue, Naked Amanda, Nayland Blake, Nightshades, Reagan Porter, Scotty Thomson, Spiral, Walkyrie, and Yandy. Thank you all for your time, energy, love, portable fans, bound burrito eating, aerial book binding, and confidence. Thanks also goes to James Mogul who granted permission use of the image of Kumi Monster suspended in my ropes (with wax being poured on her head) at the Portland Fetish Ball— the one image in this book not shot by RiggerJay.

We could not have made the project happen without the beautiful rope featured in the book. RopeExtremes.com provided all of the MFP, nylon and paracord throughout the book, and Bill came out to help with unrigging for a shoot as well. Marrow at BindMe.nl shared the beautiful jute used liberally throughout the text. Our other rope providers were ButterflyRope.com (silk and bamboo), VenusRopes.com (nylon), VintageRope.com (cotton and hemp), and SerenityBound.com (8mm green jute). Thank you for your generosity, and keep on making beautiful rope for the perverts in need.

Bondage practitioners, new and old, deserve profound passion, intention, connection, and magic. My hope is that this project will plant some seeds towards that goal of helping all of us find more joy and beauty in our lives. I am not the only bondage artist or passionate pervert who believes this is the case. I have allies in rope and erotic authenticity who are passionate about connection and rope alike, and encouraged me to put some more kink excellence out into the world in the form of this project. Thus, thanks go out to Ahleah, Aiden Fyre, Asrik Tashlin, Ayem Willing, BendYogaGirl, Boss Bondage, Christopher Angelo, Darrell Lynn, David Wraith, Deborah Addington, Diamond Blue, Dylan Richards, Esinem, Freya, Graydancer, JD of Two Knotty Boys, Jim Duvall, Karri, Lord Percival, MikeBDSM, Mitch, Monique, Murphy Blue, RiggerJay, Ruth Addams, Scotty Thomson, Sophia Sky, Suzanne SxySadist, Trialsinner, Zamil... and many others. Thank you all for demanding for excellence in kink and in me.

I am also grateful to the Western Massachusetts Bondage Group who took the first crack at test running the ties in this book as well as all of the folks who proofread the project over the years. There is something hilarious to me about rope bondage PowerPoint presentations, but y'all made it worth doing. The enthusiasm of all of my readers and feedback fans helped make the long hours worth it... even if that feedback sometimes led to further long hours :)

To my layout editor and cover designer Rob River—you always blow me away with your precision and energy, thank you for sticking with me through another project. We did it! Roxy (perfectly_bound), my fantastic copy editor—beautiful gifts come wrapped in ridiculous packages, and finding you was truly a ridiculous situation... but it led to finding your awesomeness of which I cannot say enough thanks for. Nannette H.— your last-minute eyes on this project and into my life were such a breath of fresh air. To my venue hosts, Klawdya Rothschild, RiggerJay, House Valente, and Ramblewood Retreat—thank you for taking in a wandering writer and showing me not only hospitality, but love. My thanks and love go out as well to Monique, my beautiful Butterfly—for reading text while watching Alias, breaking into hidden pools during breaks, and holding space for my journey during all of this—you are amazing.

This project is also possible thanks to everyone involved with our Indiegogo fundraising for bringing this from a dream out into the world. Phreak shot a lovely video, and Jenna Leatherman stepped in to edit it—Jenna, I owe you tacos. The world of social media spread the message around the world and helped bring supporters of all stripes together—thank you one and all. My fans and students, you continue to blow me away, it is such a blessing to be given this opportunity.

To my parents who pushed me as a child to make the world a better place—I am grateful. To my spiritual guide in all of this Work, Mother Bear—I am blessed beyond measure for the doorways we continue to open. And to everyone who continues to inspire me with their passion and artistry—I am delighted to be sharing the road with you.

Love, intention, connection, passion... here is a toast to "More."

Yours in Passion and Soul,

Lee Harrington
Anchorage, Alaska, USA
December 2014

About the Author

Lee Harrington is an internationally known spiritual and erotic authenticity educator, gender explorer, eclectic artist and award-winning author and editor on human erotic and sacred experience. He is a nice guy with a disarmingly down to earth approach to the fact that we are each beautifully complex ecosystems, and we deserve to examine the human experience from that lens. He's been traveling the globe (from Seattle to Sydney, Berlin to Boston), teaching and talking about sexuality, psychology, faith, desire and more, and is grateful for the journeys and love he has found along the way. He has been an academic and a female adult film performer, a world-class sexual adventurer, a published fetish photographer, an outspoken philosopher, a kink/bondage expert, and has been blogging about sex and spirituality since 1998.

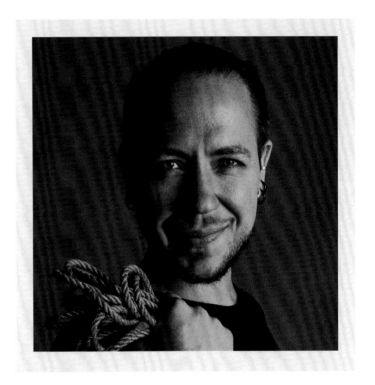

His books include *More Shibari You Can Use: Passionate Rope Bondage and Intimate Connection*, *Playing Well With Others: Your Guide to Discovering, Exploring and Negotiating the Kink, Leather and BDSM Communities* (with Mollena Williams), *Sacred Kink: The Eightfold Paths of BDSM and Beyond*, *Shibari You Can Use: Japanese Rope Bondage and Erotic Macramé*, the *Toybag Guide to Age Play*, *On Starry Thighs: Sacred and Sensual Poetry*, and *Shed Skins: Journeying in Self-Portraits*. He has also worked as an anthology editor on such projects as *Rope, Bondage, and Power* and *Spirit of Desire: Personal Explorations of Sacred Kink*, while contributing actively to other anthologies, magazines, blogs, and collaborations.

Check out the trouble Lee has been getting into, as well as his regular podcast, tour schedule, free essays, videos, coaching, and more at **www.PassionAndSoul.com**.

About the Photographer and Collaboration

By RopeRaiden and Twisted Phoenix

We first met RiggerJay online when he emailed us asking us a bunch of great questions about our ties and pictures. He came out to Detroit in fall of 2007 to take pictures of us and learn for the weekend. This was his first experience seeing Shibari-inspired suspension and from there he became a student of Japanese-inspired rope bondage. The pictures he took of us that weekend are still some of our most treasured pictures ever taken! Needless to say, a very close and dear friendship has transpired.

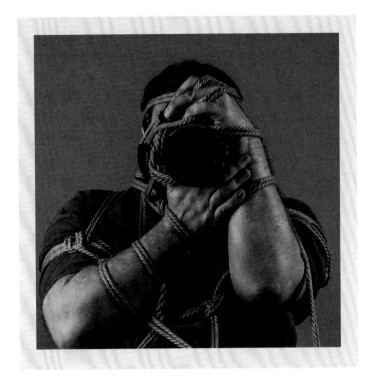

After this first meeting, we told him to attend Shibaricon with us to experience even more. It was at this event RiggerJay met Lee Harrington. Eventually, he would take private lessons with Lee and they became friends. This inspired RiggerJay to use his photography skills to capture the intimacy and artistry of Shibari in all its forms. He finds the intertwining of the artistry and technical aspects of both rope and photography fascinating and fulfilling.

One of the most interesting connections about this collaboration between RiggerJay and Lee is that the original book, *Shibari You Can Use* was the first book Rigger Jay ever bought on the subject of Shibari, it was in his hands when we first met him. In 2013, RiggerJay's skill and passion were used to re-shoot the pictures for the revised version of that same book. Now, his photography is in book two of this series as well. RiggerJay can be found today sharing his rope and photography skills at many different events in the US and Canada. Centered in New England, his efforts have led to many rope groups forming and spreading his philosophy of "Watch—Read—Learn, then make it your own."

You can see more of RiggerJay's work at **www.RiggerJay.com** and **RiggerJay.tumblr.com**.